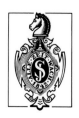

K. Mori (Ed.)

MRI of the Central Nervous System

A Pathology Atlas

With the Collaboration of
M. Kurisaka A. Moriki A. Sawada

With 116 Case Studies and 372 Figures

Springer-Verlag
Tokyo Berlin Heidelberg
New York London Paris
Hong Kong Barcelona

KOREAKI MORI, M.D., D.M.Sc.
Department of Neurosurgery, Kochi Medical School
Kohasu, Okoh-cho, Nankoku, Kochi, 783 Japan

MASAHIRO KURISAKA, M.D., D.M.Sc.
AKIHITO MORIKI, M.D., D.M.Sc.
Department of Neurosurgery, Kochi Medical School

AKIHIRO SAWADA, M.D.
Department of Radiology, Kochi Medical School

ISBN 4-431-70069-2 Springer-Verlag Tokyo Berlin Heidelberg New York
ISBN 3-540-70069-2 Springer-Verlag Berlin Heidelberg New York Tokyo
ISBN 0-387-70069-2 Springer-Verlag New York Heidelberg Berlin Tokyo

Library of Congress Cataloging-in-Publication Data

Chūsū shinkeikei shikkan no MRI. English.
MRI of the central nervous system: a pathology atlas / K. Mori (ed.)... [et al.].... p.   cm.
Translation of: Chūsū shinkeikei shikkan no MRI. Includes bibliographical references and index.
ISBN 4-431-70069-2 (hardcover) — ISBN 3-540-70069-2 (hardcover) — ISBN 0-387-70069-2
(hardcover). 1. Central nervous system — Magnetic resonance imaging — Atlases. 2. Central
nervous system — Diseases — Atlases. I. Mori, Koreaki. II. Title. [DNLM: 1. Central Nervous
System — pathology — atlases. 2. Central Nervous System Diseases — diagnosis — atlases.
3. Magnetic Resonance Imaging — atlases. WL 17 C564] RC361.C4813 1990 616.8'047548 —
dc20 DNLM/DLC for Library of Congress 90-10432 CIP

Typesetting: Koford Prints Pte Ltd., Singapore
Printing and Binding: Sambi Printing, Tokyo

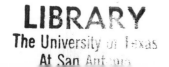

Preface

There has been great enthusiasm in the use of computerized tomography (CT) in the diagnosis of neurological disorders. However, more than 10 years have elapsed since its introduction, and it is becoming increasingly obvious that CT is not always the most effective method of investigation.

As a result of progress in computer technology, various methods of neuro-imaging have come into existence. One type in current use is magnetic resonance imaging (MRI). Soon after its introduction, it was discovered that alterations in pulse sequences resulted in significant changes in the images, and this was considered disadvantageous at the time. The difficulties in obtaining more information from MRI than from CT delayed its becoming well established as a clinical procedure.

Recently, various new and effective techniques in MRI have emerged: with the introduction of pulse sequences, it is now possible to obtain information from MRI which it was previously impossible to obtain using a CT scan alone. Realization of this has led to the establishment of this new technology in many institutions. Changes in images resulting from alterations in the pulse sequences facilitate tissue characterization which, in turn, enhance the differentiation of lesions that could not previously be diagnosed. In the past, CT was the first choice among diagnostic measures for neurological diseases, and MRI was considered to be a supplementary test, filling in for what was lacking in CT. However, with the introduction of an ever increasing number of devices, MRI is being used routinely, and it is possible that eventually CT will become supplementary to MRI.

This guide to the practical use of MRI has been compiled bearing these considerations in mind. Minimal working knowledge of the simple operations—that does not necessarily involve details in the techniques of creating television images—is all that is required in order to obtain information from the views. Thus, even if a clinician is not thoroughly familiar with the theories of MRI, he can use it as efficiently as he does the CT scan. In this book, the theoretical aspects of the principles of MRI are deliberately simplified and the text can be used solely as an atlas. In the introduction, useful general features of MRI interpretation are described and itemized, and major diseases of the central nervous system are presented.

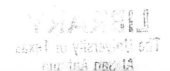

The diagnosis of neurological diseases is made primarily by the neuroradiologist, neurosurgeon, and neurologist. Some conditions are operable by the neurosurgeon whereupon it is possible to confirm the diagnoses. This book is the product of cooperation between a neuroradiologist and a neurosurgeon.

We wish to express our deep appreciation to Dr. Hiroto Kusunose, Head of Kusunose Hospital, who introduced the Hitachi G-50 MRI imaging system and made it possible to obtain the MRI films of many of these cases; to Professor Tomoho Maeda, Head of the Department of Radiology, Kochi Medical School, who encouraged us to publish the book, and to Dr. Patrick Eghwrudjakpor, a research fellow in the Department of Neurosurgery, Kochi Medical School, who proofread the English text.

December, 1990   Koreaki Mori

MRI Specifications in this Book

The magnetic resonance (MR) machine used in most of the cases is the superconductive-type Hitachi 0.5T. The pulse sequences used are: T_1 weighted image (T_1) of saturation recovery (SR) with repetition time (TR) of 500 ms and echo time (TE) of 20 ms (SR 500/20); T_2 weighted spin echo (SE) image (T_2) with TR=2000 ms, TE=60 ms (SE 2000/60) and TE=120 ms (SE 2000/40) and TE=120 ms (2000/120) and TR=1500 ms, TE=40 ms (1500/40) and TE=100 ms (SE 1500/100) for the spine.

The slice thickness is 10 mm; the matrix for reconstruction is 256 × 256; two repetitions were used and the imaging time per scan (7–10 slices) was about 7 min at TR 500 ms, 15 min at TR 1500 ms and 20 min at TR 2000 ms.

The planes of tomography are axial, coronal, and sagittal. From the choice of images, the ones useful for diagnosis for each particular case are indicated in the text. The contrast medium used for enhancement is Gd-DTPA (0.2 ml/kg).

Signal intensity is expressed as "high" intensity if it is higher than that of normal white matter, "iso" intensity if it is equivalent, and "low" intensity if it is lower.

CT scans were made primarily with GE 8600 and GE 9800 scanners. The sections are mostly axial, or coronal when indicated. An enhanced CT is shown together with a plain CT when the additional information is necessary.

Contents

General Description

1 Introduction

CT is routinely used in the investigation of diseases of the central nervous system (CNS). Its defects, however, became apparent along with its merits. Some of the defects of CT include:

1. It is sometimes not possible to differentiate between brain tumor and normal brain material, or to clearly identify the boundary of a perifocal edema.
2. The relationship between tumor, skull base, and tentorium cerebelli can often not be clearly defined.
3. The presence of artifacts may make it impossible to visualize posterior fossa tumors.
4. There is an accumulation of irradiation due to repeated follow-up examinations.

Because the boundary between gray and white matter is quite distinct on MRI, the cranial nerves, basal ganglia, brainstem nuclei, and other structures can be easily identified. Thus, for the purpose of understanding neuroanatomy, MRI is far more useful than CT.

Consequently, there are certain situations in which MRI may be considered as the examination of choice. They include:

1. Screening of patients suspected of having an intracranial tumor prior to performing any other diagnostic tests.
2. Persistence of clinical symptoms even in the absence of positive CT findings, particularly when a posterior fossa tumor is suspected.
3. Diagnosis of lesions of the white matter, including demyelination diseases and encephalitis, as well as early hemorrhage, infarction, small lesions concealed by bony structures (such as pituitary adenomas and acoustic neurinomas), atrophic lesions as in Alzheimer's disease, and estimation of the age of a hematoma.
4. Detection of multiple lesions that are similar to metastatic brain tumors, such as multiple sclerosis, multiple infarction, and others.
5. Diagnosis of spinal and spinal cord lesions where it is clearly superior to CT.

Even if MRI becomes a routine first-line investigative procedure, under the following circumstances, CT is still considered necessary:

1. If no abnormality is seen on MRI in spite of the persistence of clinical symptoms, CT is indicated in order to rule out small tumors.
2. In acute cases such as trauma, CT is preferable, and MRI, because of its long examination time, should be reserved for subacute and chronic cases.
3. CT is clearly superior in the detection of calcifications, cerebrospinal fluid (CSF) dissemination of brain tumors, etc.
4. MRI is contraindicated in patients with aneurysm clips and in those carrying pacemakers and other life support systems.

2 Principles of Imaging

Nuclear magnetic resonance (NMR) is a phenomenon which has been used for chemical analysis. Recently, extension of its application to living tissues has made it possible to diagnose diseases of the central nervous system and measure energy metabolism.

Atomic nuclei, because of their positive charges, produce magnetic fields by turning like tops and thus act like small magnets. When these nuclear magnets are introduced into a magnetic field, most of them will turn in the direction of the field; some of them will reverse, however, and the poles will turn in the direction opposite to that of the static magnetic field. If a high frequency magnetic field with a frequency equal to that of the precision is simultaneously applied to the atomic nuclei, they absorb electromagnetic waves and become energized in a manner similar to the increase in amplitude that results when external force is applied to a pendulum with the correct frequency.

This phenomenon is called the "resonance phenomenon". With the discontinuation of the high frequency magnetic field, the atomic nuclei will radiate energy and revert to their previous state. In the process, they radiate electromagnetic waves (NMR signals) whose frequencies are determined by the strength of the magnetic field and the nature of the atomic nuclei. In MRI, the NMR signals are generated by exciting the proton (^{1}H) contained in the water of the human body, and appear as an image.

NMR parameters of spin density and relaxation time are also shown as an image. "Relaxation time" refers to the time that is required for the nuclear magnets to return to their original state after the high frequency magnetic field is discontinued. There are two types of relaxation time: the first is termed T_1 (spin-lattice relaxation) and represents the time required for all the reversed nuclear magnets to revert to the field conditions in which they were prior to the application of the high frequency magnetic field. That is, it is the time required to finish radiating the energy obtained from the high frequency magnetic field into the surroundings.

The other type, T_2 (spin-spin relaxation time), represents the time required for the nuclear magnets to return from their spinning movement which started as a result of the application of the high-energy magnetic field to their original scattering movements after removal of the field. Data on tissue characteristics of the lesion can then be obtained, since some of the atomic molecular composition of the tissues and the combined condition of atomic nuclei can be calculated by correlating relaxation time with the NMR.

MRI adopts the two-dimensional Fourier transformation zeugmatography technique, which is almost the same image reconstruction technique as that used in X-ray CT. It shows the intensity of the NMR signals obtained from the differences in density of the atomic nuclei and T_1 and T_2 relaxation times in light and shade. Altogether different images are obtained depending on values chosen for TE, TR, etc. MRI has various characteristics which are supplementary to those of the X-ray CT.

MRI has no harmful effect on living tissues because of the very small quantity of energy absorbed, and it obviates the need for X-rays. Each scan takes 5–20 min. Additionally, simultaneous multiplanar tomographic scans are also possible, and white and gray matter can be clearly distinguished. MRI can produce images of the pituitary gland and posterior fossa as well as of the spinal cord without injection of a contrast agent. It is also possible to obtain a sagittal tomogram, which is difficult with X-ray CT. MRI can make it possible to diagnose cerebral infarction earlier than X-ray CT because changes in relaxation time precede organic changes.

3 MRI Anatomy

Since the most useful information that MRI provides is anatomical, understanding of anatomy is essential in the interpretation of MR images. For clinicians, it is not absolutely compulsory to possess detailed knowledge of the workings of MRI, or even of its basic principles. Since MRI is able to produce multiplanar tomograms, a three-dimensional understanding of anatomy is necessary. For this reason, MR images of the head in horizontal, sagittal, and coronal planes are presented together with corresponding schematic diagrams in this book, and sagittal sections and their schemata are shown for spinal MRI.

In general, because the T_1 weighted images show anatomical structures so well, they are presented in all three planes in this book. Only the axial image of T_2 is presented, being more sensitive in the detection of pathological lesions than the T_1 weighted image.

MRI demonstrates the cerebral sulci better than CT, making intracranial anatomy more easily understood. Structures which are surrounded by bony structures, such as the pituitary gland, brainstem, and spinal cord, are also well visualized by MRI.

Cerebrospinal fluid, having a long T_1 value, is shown as a low signal intensity (dark image) in the T_1 weighted image. Structures with signal intensities higher than that of cerebrospinal fluid are therefore clearly delineated. Since the majority of pathological lesions have long T_1 values, they usually appear as low intensities. Consequently, care must be taken not to miss them in low signal intensity areas.

In the T_2 weighted image, anatomical structures such as the corpus callosum and brainstem which have T_2 values shorter than those of neighboring structures are clearly demonstrated. Lesions with prolonged T_2 values appear whiter (high signal intensity) than surrounding tissues, and can therefore be easily detected.

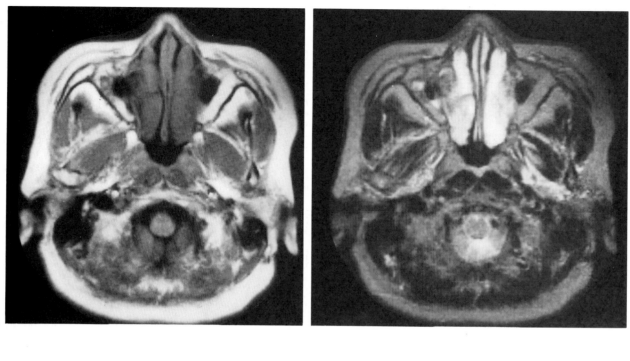

a   b

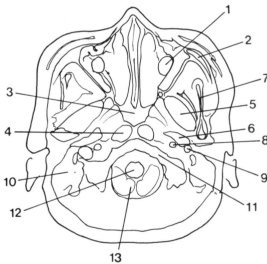

1. Maxillary sinus
2. Zygomatic arch
3. Nasopharynx
4. Internal carotid artery
5. Lateral pterygoid muscle
6. Parapharyngeal space
7. Internal jugular vein
8. Mastoid process
9. Longus capitis and colli muscles
10. Mandible
11. Occipital condyle
12. Junction of medulla and spinal cord
13. Cerebellar tonsil

Fig. 3.1. Axial image at the level of craniovertebral junction: The medullospinal junction and cerebellar tonsils are seen. **a** T₁ weighted image; **b** T₂ weighted image

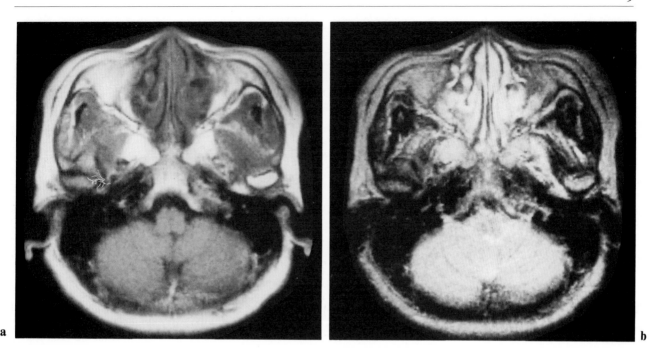

a   b

1. Medulla
2. Clivus
3. Lateral pterygoid muscle

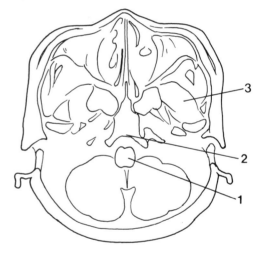

Fig. 3.2. Axial image at the level of the medulla: The clivus is shown as a high intensity area ventral to the medulla. **a** T$_1$ weighted image; **b** T$_2$ weighted image

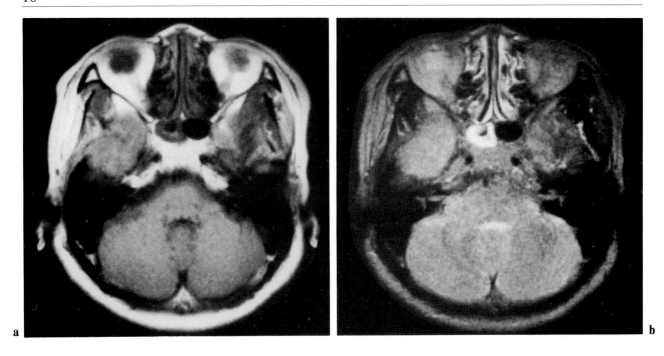

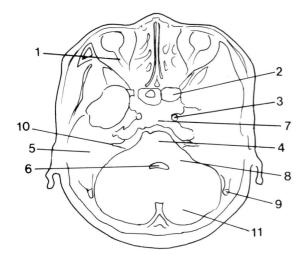

1. Optic nerve
2. Sphenoid sinus
3. Internal carotid artery
4. Pons
5. Petrous pyramid
6. Fourth ventricle
7. Clivus
8. Middle cerebellar peduncle
9. Sigmoid sinus
10. VIIth and VIIIth cranial nerves
11. Cerebellar hemisphere

Fig. 3.3. The facial and acoustic nerves can be seen at the level of the lower pons. The clivus is shown as a high intensity in the T_2 weighted image because of the fatty content of its marrow, and as a low to iso signal intensity in the T_2 weighted image. **a** T_1 weighted image; **b** T_2 weighted image

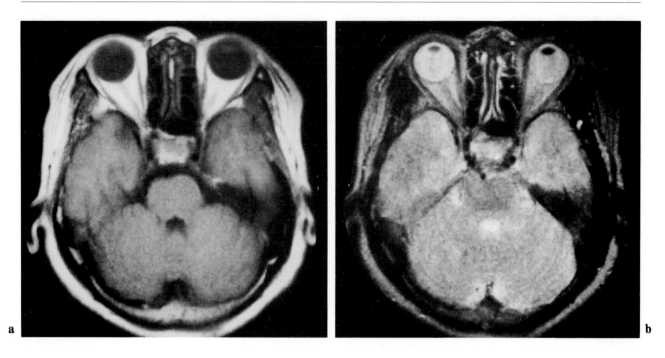

1. Internal carotid artery
2. Eyeball
3. Optic nerve
4. Pituitary gland
5. Dorsum sellae
6. Pontine tegmentum
7. Fourth ventricle
8. Vermis
9. Temporal lobe
10. Basilar artery
11. Ethmoid sinus

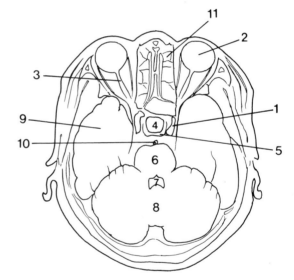

Fig. 3.4. In the T_1 weighted image, the optic nerve and orbital muscles can be seen relatively clearly because the intraorbital fat is depicted as a high signal intensity. The internal carotid artery siphon is shown as a signal void area. The outlines of the pons, fourth ventricle, cerebellum, and other parts of the brain can be clearly recognized. **a** T_1 weighted image; **b** T_2 weighted image

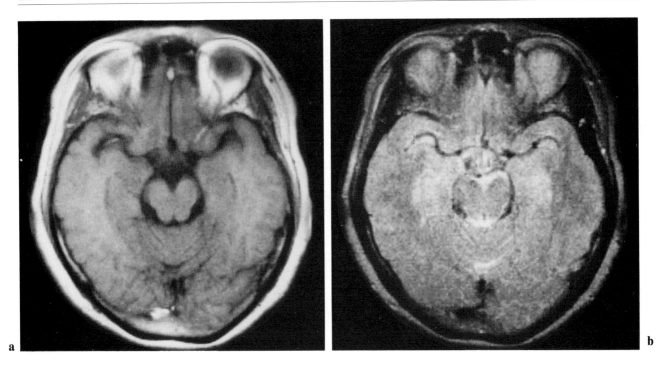

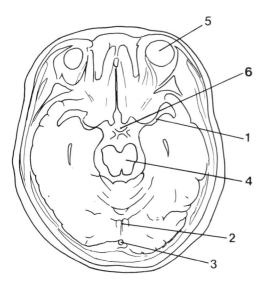

1. Middle cerebral artery
2. Straight sinus
3. Superior sagittal sinus
4. Midbrain
5. Eyeball
6. Optic chiasm

Fig. 3.5. Lower midbrain. The middle cerebral artery is shown as a signal void area because of its rapid blood flow. **a** T_1 weighted image; **b** T_2 weighted image

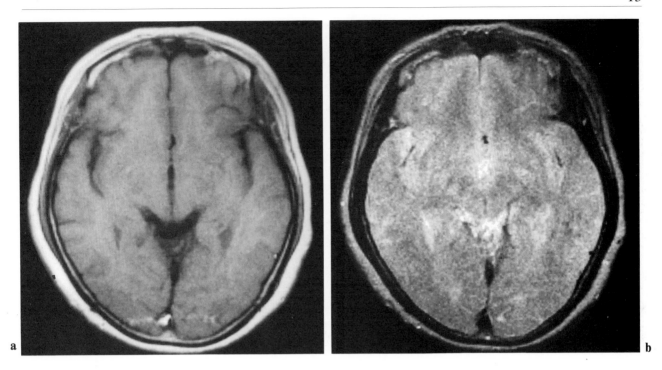

1. Interhemispheric fissure
2. Sylvian fissure
3. Third ventricle
4. Quadrigeminal cistern
5. Phase-encoding artifact
6. Occipital lobe
7. Red nucleus
8. Substantia nigra

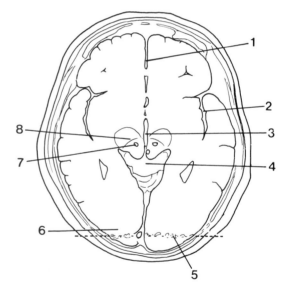

Fig. 3.6. At the level of the upper midbrain, the red nucleus and substantia nigra are seen as low signal intensity areas in the T_2 weighted image. This is believed to be due to the higher content of iron deposits found in these areas. **a** T_1 weighted image; **b** T_2 weighted image

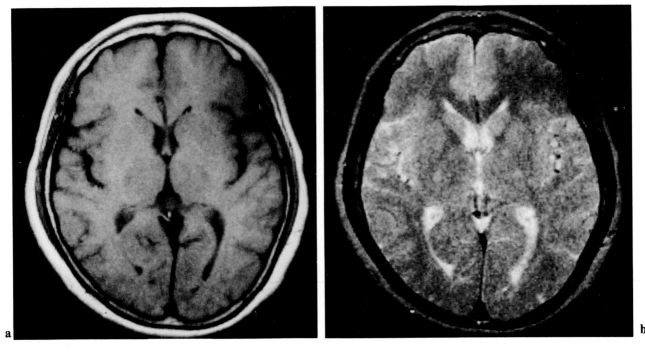

a   b

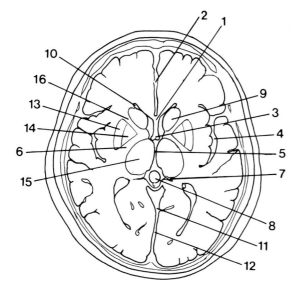

1. Genu of corpus callosum
2. Interhemispheric fissure
3. Column of fornix and anterior commissure
4. Sylvian fissure
5. Third ventricle
6. Posterior limb of internal capsule
7. Retrothalamic cistern
8. Pineal body
9. Head of caudate nucleus
10. Frontal horn
11. Straight sinus
12. Posterior falx
13. Putamen
14. Globus pallidus
15. Thalamus
16. Anterior limb of internal capsule

Fig. 3.7. The head of the caudate nucleus, putamen, globus pallidus, thalamus, internal capsule, and other parts of the brain can be seen in the basal ganglia. **a** T$_1$ weighted image; **b** T$_2$ weighted image

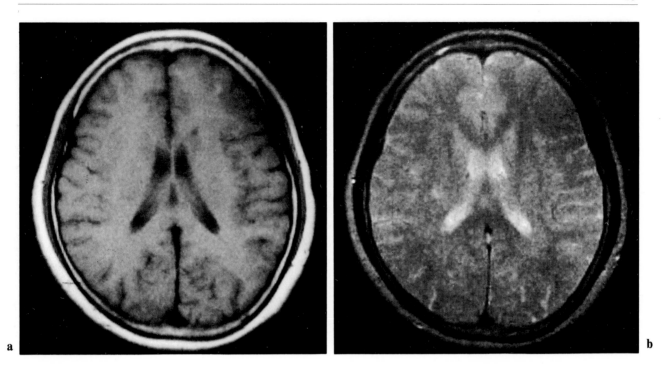

1. Temporal muscle
2. Centrum semiovale
3. Lateral ventricle
4. Splenium of corpus callosum
5. Caudate nucleus

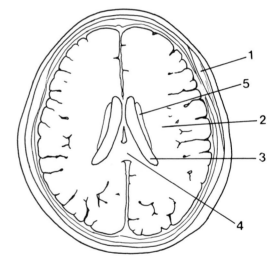

Fig. 3.8. The body of the caudate nucleus can be seen as a narrow area lateral to the lateral ventricle. It is important that care be taken not to confuse this with changes caused by demyelination. **a** T_1 weighted image; **b** T_2 weighted image

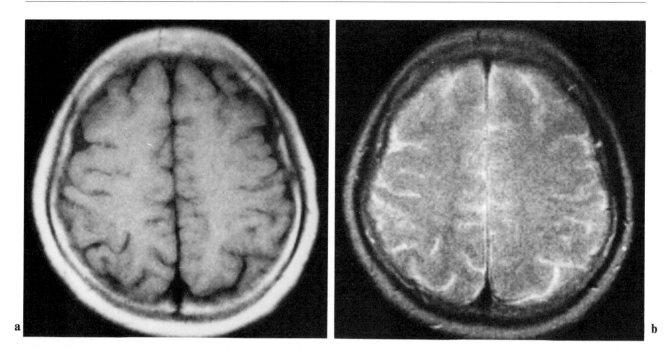

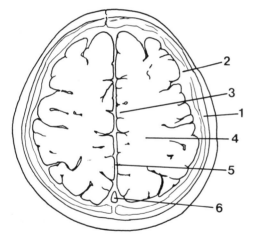

1. Temporal muscle
2. Coronal suture
3. Cingulate gyrus
4. Centrum semiovale
5. Falx cerebri
6. Superior sagittal sinus

Fig. 3.9. The centrum semiovale is seen largely as white matter lying above the corpus callosum in the horizontal sections. Its name is derived from its semiovoid shape. **a** T_1 weighted image; **b** T_2 weighted image

1. Superior sagittal sinus
2. Frontal horn
3. Interhemispheric fissure
4. Intracavernous portion of the internal carotid artery
5. Optic chiasm
6. Sylvian fissure
7. Pituitary gland
8. Sphenoid sinus
9. Zygomatic arch
10. Nasopharynx
11. Lateral pterygoid muscle
12. Medial pterygoid muscle
13. Mandible
14. Tongue
15. Pituitary stalk
16. Corpus callosum

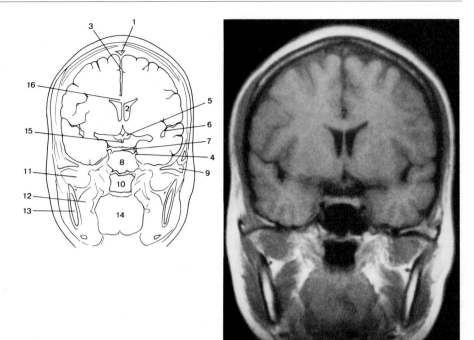

Fig. 3.10. The corpus callosum runs alongside the upper lateral ventricle. The optic chiasm, pituitary stalk, and pituitary gland can be seen beneath the thalamus. The internal carotid artery siphon can be seen on both sides of the pituitary gland

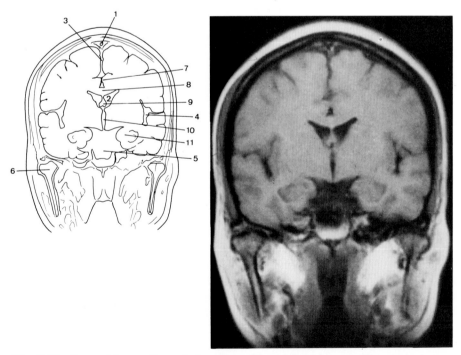

1. Superior sagittal sinus
2. Frontal horn
3. Interhemispheric fissure
4. Sylvian fissure
5. Sphenoid sinus
6. Mandible
7. Cingulate gyrus
8. Corpus callosum
9. Fornix
10. Third ventricle
11. Uncus

Fig. 3.11. Coronal image through the uncus (T_1 weighted image): The uncus is seen in the medial portion of the base of the brain

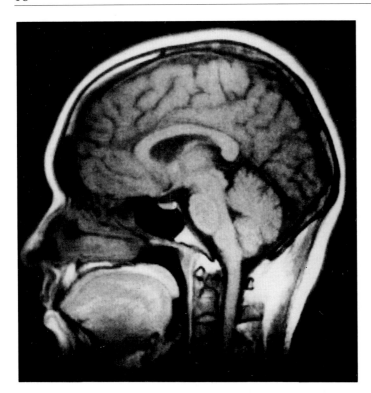

1. Corpus callosum
2. Cingulate gyrus
3. Fornix
4. Thalamus
5. Suprasellar cistern
6. Aqueduct
7. Clivus
8. Cerebellum
9. Posterior arch of C1
10. Septum pellucidum
11. Anterior commissure
12. Optic chiasm
13. Pituitary gland — anterior lobe
14. Pituitary gland — posterior lobe
15. Fourth ventricle
16. Pons
17. Anterior arch of C1
18. Cisterna magna
19. Mamillary body
20. Midbrain
21. Medulla oblongata
22. Tectum
23. Pituitary stalk
24. Superior sagittal sinus
25. Subcutaneous fatty tissue
26. Outer table
27. Diploe
28. Inner table

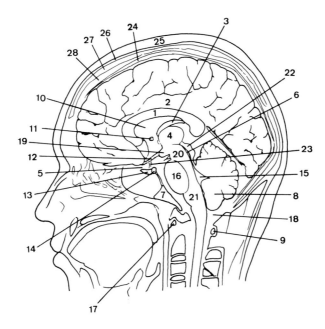

Fig. 3.12. The midline sagittal image is particularly useful in the correlation between lesions and the corpus callosum, fornix, brainstem and cerebellum. In the T_1 weighted image, the posterior lobe of the pituitary is shown as a high signal intensity and can therefore be differentiated from the anterior lobe. The pituitary stalk runs upward from the gland to the optic chiasm above. The third ventricle cannot be recognized because of partial volume effect. The thalamus which forms the lateral wall of the third ventricle is often seen on MRI. Both the aqueduct and fourth ventricle which extend from the third ventricle are always well displayed

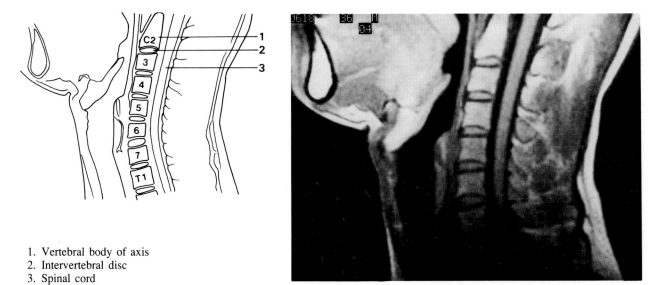

1. Vertebral body of axis
2. Intervertebral disc
3. Spinal cord

Fig. 3.13. The relationship between the vertebral body, intervertebral disc, and spinal cord can be readily understood from the sagittal image of the spine. The iso intensity of the vertebral body is due to its marrow: the body itself cannot be seen on MRI. Care should be taken not to confuse the yellow degeneration of the bone marrow for a lesion. Additionally, it should be noted that the bony spur which complicates cervical spondylosis cannot be properly demonstrated by MRI

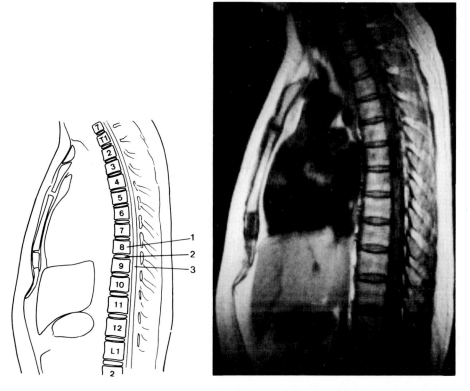

1. Vertebral body
2. Intervertebral disc
3. Spinal cord

Fig. 3.14. To obtain thoracic vertebral images, synchronization with electrocardiography is necessary to avoid phase-encoding artifacts

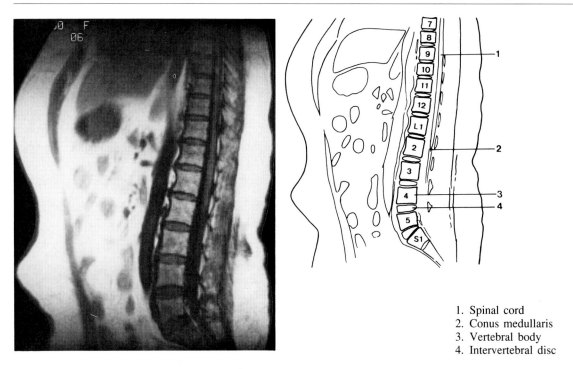

1. Spinal cord
2. Conus medullaris
3. Vertebral body
4. Intervertebral disc

Fig. 3.15. In the midline sagittal image of the lumbar spine, the relationship between the vertebral body, intervertebral disc, and spinal cord can be clearly seen. The conus medullaris of adults is usually located at the level of the second lumbar vertebral body

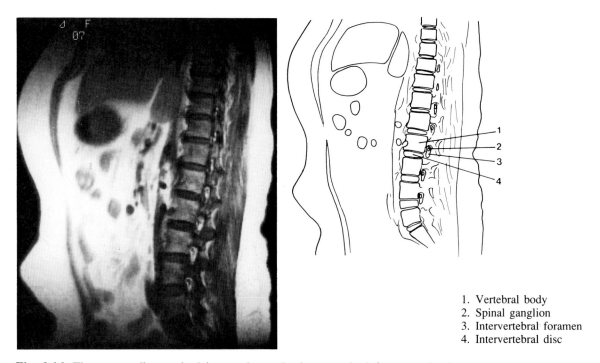

1. Vertebral body
2. Spinal ganglion
3. Intervertebral foramen
4. Intervertebral disc

Fig. 3.16. The paramedian sagittal image shows the intervertebral foramen clearly because of the contrast with the paravertebral fatty tissue. The spinal ganglia and nerve roots are dark against the bright fatty tissue. Images of this section are useful in cases of suspected lumbar disc hernia

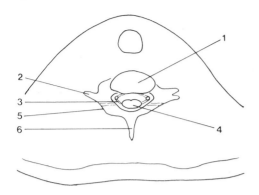

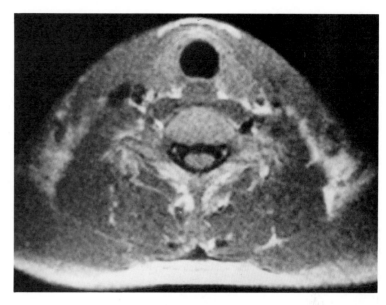

1. Vertebral body
2. Transverse process
3. Spinal nerve roots
4. Spinal cord
5. Facet joint
6. Spinous process

Fig. 3.17. Axial image of the cervical spine (T$_1$ weighted image): The spinal cord is shown more clearly than on CT

4 Abnormal Findings in MRI

The MRI signal intensity is influenced by the following factors:

1. Proton density (ρ)
2. T_1 relaxation time
3. T_2 relaxation time
4. Flow speed

Proton density is very low in both air and compact bone but is high in the cerebrospinal fluid. The contrast on MRI between soft tissues and structures of the brain parenchyma, however, is determined primarily by T_1 and T_2. The T_1 and T_2 characteristics of each tissue are shown in Table 4.1.

Table 4.1. Signal intensity of tissue

T_1 weighted image			T_2 weighted image		
T_1	Signal intensity	Tissue	T_2	Signal intensity	Tissue
Short	High	Fat	Short	Low	Muscle
↑	Slightly high	White matter	↑	Slightly low	White matter
	Slightly low	Gray matter		Slightly high	Gray matter
	Slightly low	Muscle		Slightly high	Fat
↓	Low	CSF	↓		
Long	Low	Bone cortex	Long	High	CSF

Prolongation of T_1 lowers the signal intensity (dark), while prolongation of T_2 creates a high signal intensity (bright). In the T_1 weighted image, the white matter is shown as white and the gray matter looks slightly dark, as they appear macroscopically. This pattern is reversed in the T_2 weighted image. On the other hand, CSF is dark in the T_1 weighted image but bright in the T_2 weighted image. Fat appears bright in the T_1 weighted image, but slightly dark in T_2 weighted image. Compared to normal tissues, most lesions (including tumors, edemas, degenerations, necroses, inflammations, and cysts) prolong both T_1 and T_2 (Fig. 4.1). The classification of tissues and lesions according to their signal intensity patterns is shown in Table 4.2. The signal intensity changes occurring in hematomas reflect chronological changes of hemoglobin (Table 4.3). Blood is usually shown as a complete absence of signal when the flow is rapid. It may, however, be shown as high signal intensity when the flow is slow, the latter being due to a phenomenon of paradoxical enhancement.

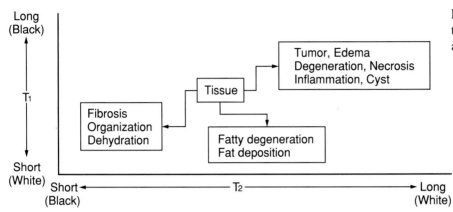

Fig. 4.1. The relationship between the T_1 and T_2 values for each tissue and disease

Table 4.2. MRI signal intensity of tissue and lesion in T_1 and T_2 weighted images

	T_1	T_2	
1	High	Low	Fat, subacute hematoma (with some exceptions), melanoma (with some exception)
2	High	High	Chronic hematoma, high proteinaceous cyst, venous sinus obstruction
3	Low	Low	Muscle, meningioma (with some exceptions), acute hematoma
4	Low	High	Neoplasm, ischemia, edema, demyelination, inflammation, fluid, cyst
5	Very low	Very low	Calcium, high blood flow, air, hemosiderin, paramagnetic substance

Table 4.3. MRI changes of hematoma with time

Stage (age)	Composition	Signal intensity	
		T_1	T_2
Acute (1 – 4 days)	Deoxyhemoglobin	Low	Low
Subacute (5 – 12 days)	Intracellular methemoglobin	High	Low
Chronic (2 weeks – 1.5 years)	Extracellular methemoglobin	High	High
Old (6 months – 5 years)	Residual methemoglobin, CSF, gliosis	Low	High
Old (5 days – several years)	Hemosiderin	Void	Void

Optimal pulse sequences should be selected in order to obtain T_1 and T_2 weighted images. The main pulse sequences are as follows:

SR = Saturation recovery (90°–TR) n

IR = Inversion recovery (180°–TI–90°–T') n

SE = Spin echo (90°–TE/2–180°–T') n

(TR = TI + T' or TR = TE/2 + T')

The characteristics of each of the pulse sequences are shown in Table 4.4. At present, SE is the most commonly used. Shortening of TR in SE produces a T_1 weighted image (Fig. 4.2) and the T_2 weighted image is made by prolonging TE (Fig. 4.3). Thus, in order to obtain T_1 weighted images, it is necessary to shorten both TR (<1000 ms) and TE (<30 ms). This is commonly referred to as SR. Prolongation of TR (>1500 ms) and TE (>50 ms) produces T_2 weighted images.

Table 4.4. MRI produced by different pulse sequences

	SR	IR	SE
Scanning sequence	TR = 300–500ms TE ≤ 20–40ms	TR = 1000–3000ms TI = 300–500ms	TR = 1000–3000ms TE≥50ms
Information obtained	T_1 weighted image	T_1 weighted image	T_2 weighted image
Advantages	–The parenchyma and CSF are clearly demonstrated and useful morphological information can be obtained. –Examination time is short.	–There is good contrast of white and gray matter. –It is not as sensitive as SE in demonstrating lesions, but is in discriminating edema from solid portions of tumors and demonstrating intratumoral structures. –It is also useful for demonstrating lesions in brainstem.	–The discrimination of white and gray matter is excellent, and it is useful for detecting lesions. –Multiple slices are also possible.
Disadvantages	–There is no contrast between white and gray matter. Consequently, it is inferior in the detection of lesions.	–It is difficult to discriminate between bone, CSF and air.	–Because it is difficult to discriminate parenchyma from CSF, it is inferior in obtaining intrastuctural information.

SR, saturation recovery; IR, inversion recovery; SE, spin echo; TR, repetition, time; T_1 spin-lattice relaxation; T_2, spin-spin relaxation; TI, inversion time

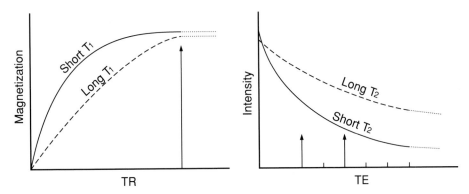

Fig. 4.2. The relationship between signal intensity of a T$_2$ weighted image and pulse sequence. If TR is sufficiently prolonged, the difference in signal intensity of T$_1$ diminishes. With sufficient prolongation of TE, however, the difference in signal intensity of T$_2$ becomes more significant. In other words, if TR and TE are prolonged, a T$_2$ weighted image can be obtained. Reproduced, with permission, from [Brant-Zawdzki M, Norman D (eds) (1987) Magnetic resonance imaging of the central nervous system. Raven Press, New York]

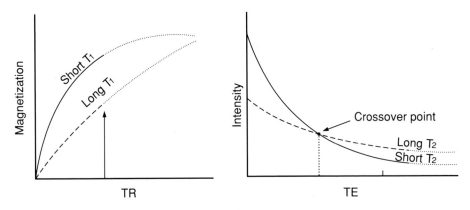

Fig. 4.3. The relationship between signal intensity of a T$_1$ weighted image and pulse sequence. At the crossover point, if T$_2$ weighted image is made, it is almost impossible to distinguish any difference in the values of T$_2$, however, TR is shortened sufficiently, differences in the values of T$_1$ will be emphasized. In other words, a T$_1$ weighted image can be obtained. Reproduced, with permission, from [Brant-Zawdzki M, Norman D (eds) (1987) Magnetic resonance imaging of the central nervous system. Raven Press, New York]

5 Predilection Sites of CNS Lesions

Most central nervous system lesions are known to have specific sites of predilection. A knowledge of lesions most frequently encountered in each location will facilitate their diagnosis on MRI.

Cerebral Lesions

Congenital Anomalies
These anomalies include malformations with anatomical defects, phakomatosis, arteriovenous malformation, and leukodystrophy.

Trauma
Hemorrhage, contusion, and swelling (edema) occur either in isolation or in association with other lesions.

Tumors
Primary tumors include glial tumors originating from glial cells, and nonglial tumors which arise from cells of nonglial origin. Metastatic tumors form the majority of secondary tumors.

Infections
These include abscesses and encephalitis.

Vascular Lesions
Hemorrhages or hematomas due to ruptured blood vessels and infarctions due to occlusion of vessels are some examples.

Miscellaneous
So-called neurological diseases, such as degenerative diseases, toxic and metabolic disorders, as well as multiple sclerosis and parasites are included here.

Extra-axial Lesions

Supratentorial space-occupying lesions are most common, with the exception of lesions of the posterior fossa and parasellar region. Epidural (or extradural) and subdural hematomas appear under the subgroup of acute hematomas. Subdural hematomas are also included in the subgroups of subacute and chronic hematomas. Other lesions found here are meningiomas, chordomas, epidermoid cysts, etc.

Intra- and Suprasellar Lesions

Intrasellar Lesions

Most intrasellar lesions are pituitary adenomas. Others which occur much less frequently include craniopharyngiomas, arachnoid cysts, endotheliomas, abscesses, Rathke's cleft cysts, and empty sellar lesions.

Suprasellar Lesions

These are common lesions and include suprasellar extension of pituitary adenomas, craniopharyngiomas, arachnoid cysts, epidermoids, germinomas, teratomas, hamartomas, and chordomas. Lateral extension of pituitary adenomas into the cavernous sinus and posterior invasion into the interpeduncular cistern may also occur. Craniopharyngiomas very often extend from the clivus and reveal bony destruction and calcification.

Posterior Fossa Lesions

Extra-axial Lesions

All subarachnoid spaces in the posterior fossa enlarge in cases of atrophy of the cerebellum and brainstem. In the former, the folia may also enlarge. Local dilatation of the subarachnoid space may be seen in cerebellopontine (CP) angle tumors or clival tumors which displace the brainstem. Other space-occupying lesions in this category include arachnoid cysts, epidermoids, acoustic neurinomas, meningiomas, basilar artery aneurysms, and chordomas.

Fourth Ventricle Tumors

Prominent among the space-occupying lesions in this region are medulloblastomas, ependymomas, choroid plexus papillomas and cystic astrocytomas. Metastatic tumors may also occur.

Cerebellar Lesions

Medulloblastomas in the mid-cerebellar region and astrocytomas in the cerebellar hemisphere are some of the common tumors. Hemangioblastomas, hemorrhages, infarctions, metastases, abscesses, etc., are also seen in the cerebellum.

Brainstem Lesions

Gliomas, hemorrhages, infarctions, and angiomas are among the most common lesions found in the brain stem.

Ventricular Lesions

The ventricular system becomes dilated in hydrocephalus and in cerebral atrophy and is compressed and deformed by space-occupying lesions. In intracerebral hemorrhages, the ventricular wall is often penetrated with resultant intraventricular hemorrhage. The choroid plexus often reveals physiological calcification, and periventricular calcification is frequently observed in toxoplasmosis and tuberous sclerosis. Meningiomas, third ventricle colloid cysts, and choroid plexus papillomas are among the major intraventricular tumors. Occasionally, extension of paraventricular tumors into the ventricle may appear as intraventricular tumors.

Among these are gliomas, malignant lymphomas, germinomas, teratomas, ependymomas, and dermoid and epidermoid tumors. Germinomas may also show intraventricular spread.

Lesions of the Subarachnoid Space

In communicating hydrocephalus, there is dilatation of the subarachnoid space proximal to the obstruction. Intracerebral tumors may also enlarge the subarachnoid space by displacement of the brainstem.

The subarachnoid space is compromised by swelling of the brain (brain edema), hydrocephalus, subdural fluid collections, brain tumors, and others. Meningeal infiltration of a brain tumor may obstruct the subarachnoid space, and ruptured aneurysms cause subarachnoid hemorrhages.

Cranial Vault Lesions

Unilateral cerebral atrophy may cause a thickening of the cranial vault with an ipsilateral enlargement of the air sinuses. Lesions that cause local thickening of the skull include fibrous dysplasias, meningiomas, osteomas, cephalhematomas, and Paget's disease. Local bone thickening often occurs in lesions which are located close to the skull, such as subarachnoid cysts and chronic subdural hematomas. In addition to bone defects due to tumors and fractures, diploic cavernous angiomas may also display bone defects. Other lesions which show such changes include bone metastases, multiple myelomas, eosinophilic granulomas, tuberculomas, cranium bifidum occultum, and sinus pericranii.

Spinal Lesions

MRI is the most useful diagnostic technique for spinal lesions, warranting a more detailed description of lesions in this location.

Spinal Tumors

Spinal tumors are classified into three types: (a) extradural tumor, (b) intradural extramedullary tumor, and (c) intramedullary tumor. Neurinomas are the most common spinal tumors, followed closely by meningiomas, which occur predominantly in the thoracic region. Both tumors often present as intradural extramedullary tumors. If metastatic tumors (which are mostly extradural) are excluded, intradural extramedullary tumors would account for most of the spinal cord tumors, followed in order of frequency by extradural and intramedullary tumors. With regard to the sites of lesions, the thoracic spine is the most frequently involved region, followed by the lumbar, cervical, and sacral regions.

The greater proportion of extradural tumors is formed by metastatic tumors which arise from primary cancers in the lung, breast, prostate, and digestive tract. The majority spread to the vertebral body, causing bone destruction and spinal cord compression. Some brain tumors, especially medulloblastomas and germinomas, may give rise to spinal metastases. Primary extradural tumors include chordomas, sarcomas, and myelomas.

Most intradural extramedullary tumors are neurinomas or meningiomas. Neurinomas account for the majority of spinal cord tumors, originating from spinal nerves and developing in a dumbbell shape inside and outside the dura, frequently passing through the intervertebral foramen (hourglass- or dumbbell-shaped tumor). When these are multiple tumors, they form part of von Recklinghausen's disease.

Gliomas account for most intramedullary tumors. Among the primary intramedullary tumors, ependymomas occur most frequently, followed by astrocytomas.

Congenital tumors such as epidermoids, dermoids and teratomas may also develop. Skin abnormalities such as dimples, nevi, and hair tufts may be observed in the midline in patients with congenital tumors. Epidermoids may be complicated by dermal sinus tracts extending towards the outer surface. Lipomas may be associated with spina bifida. It is well documented that syringomyelia is complicated by spinal cord tumors.

Vascular Disorders of the Spinal Cord

Spinal vascular disorders occur much less frequently than cerebral vascular disorders. When a spinal subarachnoid hemorrhage is present, the most probable cause is a spinal arteriovenous malformation. Most cases of extradural hemorrhage result from traumatic damage to the extradural venous plexus. Extradural hemorrhage is predisposed to occur in the thoracic vertebrae and in the transitional portion between the cervical and thoracic vertebrae, leading to a compression paraplegia within a short period of time. This hemorrhage exhibits symptoms similar to those of acute spinal extradural abscesses.

Spinal arteriovenous malformations comprise about 5% of all spinal tumors. This malformation is found mostly in the young age group, and especially in males. Since the primitive vascular plexus is present on the surface of the spinal cord, and especially since the vascular system on the posterior surface completes later, arteriovenous malformations are observed mostly in the posterior aspect of the spinal cord. About 80% are found dorsolaterally, and, in terms of levels, about 60%, 30%, and 10% are seen in the lower thoracic, upper thoracic, and cervical cords, respectively. Subarachnoid hemorrhages account for only 10% of spinal vascular disorders. Progression is gradual and deterioration occurs in stages over a relatively long period, with the chief complaint being motor dysfunction in the lower extremities. Therefore, these must be differentiated from spinal cord tumors. If primary disorders such as trauma, infection and tumor are not obvious in progressive spinal cord disorders, arteriovenous malformations should always be suspected.

The causes of spinal infarction include: (a) occlusion or stenosis of extradural vessels, (b) occlusion or stenosis of spinal vessels, and (c) systemic hypotension due to shock, cardiac arrest, etc. With regard to the sites of infarct, this disorder may be classified into: (a) transverse infarct, (b) infarct of the region of the anterior spinal artery, (c) infarct of the region of the posterior spinal artery, and (d) venous pencil-like infarction in the deep posterior funiculus.

When the anterior spinal artery is occluded, the anterior 2/3 of the spinal cord is damaged with a resultant anterior spinal artery syndrome (characterized by radicular diffuse pain, flaccid tetraplegia or paraplegia, sensory dissociation, and vesico-rectal dysfunction). The syndrome occurs at the level of the thoracic cord since this forms the border area between ascending and descending arteries. When the large radicular artery (Adamkiewicz's artery) which branches off the aorta and runs between the T9 and L2 vertebrae is occluded, an extensive infarct is formed covering the area from the lower thoracic down to the lumbosacral cord. Flaccid paralysis and dysfunction of superficial and deep sensation occur, resembling transverse impairment. Occlusion of the central artery results in damage to the posterior horn and central portion. This presents as a central artery syndrome, exhibiting lower motor neuron signs corresponding to the damaged level. When the posterior spinal artery is occluded, the posterior funiculus and posterior horn are impaired, exhibiting a posterior spinal artery syndrome; however, this is quite rare.

Spinal Cord Injuries

Most spinal cord injuries are indirect and closed injuries resulting from a strong impact on the spine. Spinal fractures and dislocations often result from hyperflexion, hyperextension, and sharp and extensive rotatory movement of the spine. Direct or open injuries include those from gunshots and stabbings. Traffic accidents account for about half of these injuries, followed by occupational and sports injuries. The thoracolumbar junction is most often involved, followed by the cervical vertebrae.

Spinal injuries range from concussions to contusions and lacerations, thus varying in severity. If accompanied by edema or hemorrhage, spinal cord injuries are considered to be severe. The most severe form is a spinal cord transection leading to spinal shock.

Spinal fractures include linear fractures, compression fractures, and fracture dislocations. In compression fractures, the posterior longitudinal ligament is not severed, making these injuries stable. Fracture dislocations are the most important clinically. They are completely unstable injuries since the posterior longitudinal ligament is severed, the axis of the spine shifts, and they are accompanied by fracture of the posterior joint including damage to the joint capsule. Among the special fractures are the Jefferson fracture (fracture of the atlas) and the Chance fracture (horizontal fracture of the lumbar vertebra due to seat belts).

Cervical Spondylosis

These are lesions caused by regression and degeneration of the cervical intervertebral discs. They are sometimes referred to as cervical osteochondroses or cervical spondylosis deformans. In about 75% of people above 50 years of age, these changes can be seen on X-rays. The disorders have a tendency to occur more often in males, and are frequently observed in the area between C4 and C7 showing lordosis (C5/6 followed by C6/7 and C4/5). Progression is gradual and onset in patients younger than 40 years of age is uncommon except where there is a history of trauma.

Herniated Intervertebral Discs

From a static point of view, the lower lumbar vertebrae are the most heavily loaded. Consequently, herniation frequently occurs in the fourth (L4) or fifth (L5) intervertebral disc. In addition to degeneration of the intervertebral discs, a variety of external forces on the back resulting from sports, occupation, and daily living activities may cause lacerations of the outer annulus fibrosus and prolapse of the inner nucleus pulposus, leading to herniation. Since the central portion of the intervertebral disc is posteriorly lined by the posterior longitudinal ligament, the nucleus pulposus protrudes into the weak areas on both sides of the ligament inclining either to the right or left.

In the lumbar vertebrae, a herniated intervertebral disc at a given level compresses the nerve root of the segments below it; thus a herniated L5 intervertebral disc would compress the nerve root of the S1 nerve. If, however, the intervertebral disc protrudes laterally and shifts upwards to the intervertebral foramen, the nerve root above it may be compressed. When the herniation is extensive, all of the descending nerve roots are affected, bilateral symptoms occur, and urinary incontinence may result. The mechanism of the occurrence of symptoms and signs varies; the symptoms fluctuate since the "ruptured disc" develops from 20–30 years of age, followed gradually by back pain and sciatica. In the 40–50 years age group, spondylosis occurs and spinal canal and nerve foramina are compressed not only anteriorly but also posteriorly and posterolaterally. Consequently, asthenia on walking develops together with back pain and numbness, while the symptoms are relieved at rest.

Other Vertebral Diseases

Herniated cervical intervertebral discs are often associated with cervical vertebral disorders, found mostly in the lower cervical vertebrae. According to the direction of the protrusion, this herniation can be divided into three forms: (a) median, (b) paramedian, and (c) lateral. The lateral form is the most frequently seen. The protruded disc compresses a nerve root one number higher than its corresponding level. Herniation of the thoracic intervertebral disc is rare. When it occurs, it is often located in the median position and may be misdiagnosed as a degenerative or demyelinating disease. Even a relatively small hernia may cause severe spinal cord damage. In a narrow cervical canal, symptoms easily develop following cervical disorders, herniated intervertebral discs, traumas, infections, etc.

In general, ossification of the posterior longitudinal ligament (OPLL) is asymptomatic and is often found incidentally on X-rays. It occurs frequently in Japanese people and involves 2 or 3 vertebrae between C3 and C6; occasionally, the spinal cord is compressed. Males are affected slightly more often than females. Ossification of the yellow ligament (OYL) occurs in the thoracic region and occasionally causes symptoms associated with cord compression.

Congenital anomalies of the craniovertebral junction include: (1) atlanto-axial dislocation (due to congenital growth defect of the transverse ligament of the atlas, aplasia, or hypoplasia of the dens, etc.), (2) Klippel-Feil syndrome, and (3) assimilation or occipitalization of the atlas.

Spinal infections include epi- and subdural empyema, myelitis, postoperative infections of the intervertebral disc space, and Pott's disease (osteomyelitis of the spine).

Bibliography

Albert A, Lee BC, Saint-Louis L, Deck MD (1986) MRI of optic chiasm and optic pathways. AJNR 7: 255–258

Anderson-Berg WT, Strand M, Lempert TE, Rosenbaum AE, Joseph PM (1986) Nuclear magnetic resonance and gamma camera tumor imaging using gadolinium-labeled monoclonal antibodies. J Nucl Med 27: 829–833

Asakura T, Uetsuhara K (1988) Advances in diagnostic and therapeutic applications of magnetic resonance imaging for CNS lesions. Brain and Nerve 40:451–459 (English abstract)

Atlas SW, Grossman RI, Hackney DB, Gomori JM, Campagna N, Goldberg HI, Bilaniuk LT, Zimmerman RA (1988) Calcified intracranial lesions: detection with gradient-echo-acquisition rapid MR imaging. AJNR 9: 253–259

Awad IA, Spetzler RF, Hodak JA, Awad CA, Williams F Jr, Carey R (1987) Incidental lesions noted on magnetic resonance imaging of the brain: prevalence and clinical significance in various age groups. Neurosurgery 20: 222–227

Axel L, Morton D (1987) MR flow imaging by velocity-compensated/uncompensated difference images. JCAT 11: 31–34

Babcock EE, Brateman L, Weinreb JC, Horner SD, Nunnally RL (1985) Edge artifacts in MR images: chemical shift effect. JCAT 9: 252–257

Bell RA (1987) Magnetic resonance instrumentation. In: Brant-Zawadzki M. Norman D (eds) Magnetic resonance imaging of the central nervous system. Raven Press, New York, pp13–22

Bellon EM, Haacke EM, Coleman PE, Sacco DC, Steiger DA, Gangarosa RE (1986) MR artifacts: a review. AJR 147: 1271–1281

Berquist TH (ed) (1987) Magnetic resonance of the musculoskeletal system. Raven Press, New York

Berry I, Brant-Zawadzki M, Osaki L, Brasch R, Murovic J, Newton TH (1986) Gd-DTPA in clinical MR of the brain: 2 extraaxial lesions and normal structures. AJR 147: 1231–1235

Bobman SA, Riederer SJ, Lee JN, Tasciyan T, Farzaneh F, Wang HZ (1986) Pulse sequence extrapolation with MR imaging synthesis. Radiology 159: 253–258

Bradley WG (1987a) Pathophysiologic correlates of signal alterations. In: Brant-Zawadzki M, Norman D (eds) Magnetic resonance imaging of the central nervous system. Raven Press, New York, pp23–42

Bradley WG (1987b) Magnetic resonance appearance of flowing blood and cerebrospinal fluid. In: Brant-Zawadzki M, Norman D (eds) Magnetic resonance imaging of the central nervous system. Raven Press, New York, pp83–96

Bradley WG, Waluch V (1985) Blood flow: Magnetic resonance imaging. Radiology 154: 443–450

Brant-Zawadzki M (1987) Magnetic resonance imaging: The bare necessities. In: Brant-Zawadzki M, Norman D (eds) Magnetic resonance imaging of the central nervous system. Raven Press, New York, pp1–12

Brant-Zawadzki M, Berry I, Osaki L, Brasch R, Murovic J, Norman D (1986a) Gd-DTPA in clinical MR of the brain: 1. intraaxial lesions; 2. extraaxial lesions. AJNR 7: 781–793

Brant-Zawadzki M, Berry M, Osaki I, Brasch R, Murovic J, Norman D (1986b) Gd-DTPA in clinical MR of the brain: 1. intraaxial lesions. AJR 147: 1223–1230

Braun IF, Malko JA, Davis PC, Hoffman JC Jr, Jacob LH (1986) The behavior of Pantopaque on MR: in vivo and in vitro analysis. AJNR 7: 997–1001

Buxton RB, Edelman RR, Rosen BR, Wismer GL, Brady TJ (1987) Contrast in rapid MR imaging: T1- and T2-weighted imaging. JCAT 11: 7–16

Buxton RB, Wismer GL, Brady TJ, Rosen BR (1986) Quantitative proton chemical shift imaging. Magn Reson Med 3: 881–900

Bydder GM, Young IR (1985a) MR imaging: clinical use of the inversion recovery sequence. JCAT 9: 659–675

Bydder GM, Young IR (1985b) Clinical use of partial saturation and saturation recovery sequence in MR imaging. JCAT 9: 1020–1032

Bydder GM, Payne JA, Collins AG, Thomas DGT, Davis CH, Cox IJ, Ross BD, Young IR (1987) Clinical use of rapid T2-weighted partial saturation sequences in MR imaging. JCAT 11: 17–23

Claussen C, Laniado M, Schorner W, Niedorf HP, Weinmann HJ, Fiegler W, Felix R (1985) Gadolinium-DTPA in MR imaging of glioblastomas and intracranial metastases. AJNR 6: 669–674

Cohen MD, McGuire W, Cory DA, Smith JA (1986) MR appearance of blood and blood products: an in vitro study. AJR 146: 1293–1297

Condon B, Patterson J, Wyper D, Hadley D, Grant R, Teasdale G, Rowan J (1986) The use of magnetic resonance imaging to measure the intracranial cerebrospinal fluid volume. Lancet 1: 1355–1357

Daniels DL, Pech P, Pojunas KW, Kilgore DP, Williams AL, Haughton VM (1986) Trigeminal nerve: anatomic correlations with MR imaging. Radiology 159: 577–583

Davis CA, Genant HK, Dunham JS (1986) The effects of bone in proton NMR relaxation times of surrounding liquids. Invest Radiol 21: 472–477

Di Chiro G, Knop RH, Girton ME, Dwyer AJ, Doppman JL, Patronas NJ, Gansow OA, Brechbiel MW, Brooks RA (1985) MR cisternography and myelography with Gd-DPTA in monkeys. Radiology 157: 373–377

Dillon WP (1986) Applications of magnetic resonance imaging to the head and neck. Sem Ultrasound 7: 202–215

Drayer B, Burger P, Darwin R, Riederer S, Herfkens R, Johnson GA (1986a) Magnetic resonance imaging of brain iron. AJNR 7: 373–380

Drayer B, Burger P, Darwin R, Riederer S, Herfkens R, Johnson GA (1986b) MRI of brain iron. AJR 147: 103–110

Dumoulin CL, Hart HR Jr (1986) Magnetic resonance angiography. Radiology 161: 717–720

Dwyer AJ, Knop RH, Hoult DI (1985) Frequency shift artifacts in MR imaging. JCAT 9: 16–18

Edelman RR, Stark DD, Saini S, Ferrucci JT Jr, Dinsmore RE, Ladd W, Brady TJ (1986) Oblique planes of section in MR imaging. Radiology 159: 807–810

Ehman RL (1985) MR imaging with surface coils. Radiology 157: 549–550

Ehman RL, Wesbey GE, Moon KL, Williams RD, McNamara MT, Couet WR, Tozer TN, Brasch RC (1985) Enhanced MRI of tumors utilizing a new nitroxyl spin label contrast agent. Magnetic Resonance Imaging 3: 89–97

Enzmann DR, Rubin JB, DeLaPaz R, Wright A (1986) Cerebrospinal fluid pulsation: benefits and pitfalls in MR imaging. Radiology 161: 773–778

Enzmann DR, Rubin JB, Wright A (1987) Use of cerebrospinal fluid gating to improve T2-weighted images, part I. The spinal cord. Radiology 162: 763–767

Feiglin DH, George CR, MacIntyre WJ, O'Donnell JK, Go RT, Pavlicek W, Meaney TF (1985) Gated cardiac magnetic resonance structural imaging: optimization by electronic axial rotation. Radiology 154: 129–132

Feinberg DA, Mills CM, Posin JP, Ortendahl DA, Hylton NM, Crooks LE, Watts JC, Kaufman L, Arakawa M (1985) Multiple spin echo magnetic resonance imaging. Radiology 155: 437–442

Felix R, Schorner W, Laniado M, Niendorf HP, Claussen C, Fiegler W, Speck U (1985) Brain tumors: MR imaging with Gadolinium-DTPA. Radiology 156: 681–688

Finn EJ, Di Chiro G, Brooks RA, Satto S (1985) Ferromagnetic materials in patients: detection before MR imaging. Radiology 156: 139–141

Fischer MR, Barker B, Amparo BG (1985) MR imaging using specialized coils. Radiology 157: 443–447

Flannigan BD, Bradley WG Jr, Mazziotta JC, Rauschning W, Bentson JR, Lufkin RB, Hieshima GB (1985) Magnetic resonance imaging of the brainstem: normal structure and basic functional anatomy. Radiology 154: 375–383

Frahm J, Haase A, Matthaei D (1986) Rapid NMR imaging using the FLASH technique. JCAT 10: 363–368

Gadian DG, Payne JA, Bryant DJ, Young IR, Carr DH, Bydder GM (1985) Gadolinium-DTPA as a contrast agent in MR imaging-theoretical projections and practical observations. JCAT 9: 242–251

Gomori JM, Grossman RI, Goldberg HI, Zimmerman RA, Bilaniuk LT (1985) Intracranial hematomas: imaging by high-field MR. Radiology 157: 87–93

Gomori JM, Grossman RI (1987) Head and neck hemorrhage. In: Kressel HY (ed) Magnetic resonance annual. Raven Press, New york, pp71–117

Haacke EM, Bearden FH, Clayton JR, Linga NR (1986) Reduction of MR imaging time by the hybrid fast-scan technique. Radiology 158: 521–529

Hackney DB, Grossman RI, Zimmerman RA, Joseph PM, Goldberg HI, Bilaniuk LT (1986) MR characteristics of iodophendylate (Pantopaque). JCAT 10: 401–403

Haughton VM, Rimm AA, Sobocinski KA, Papke RA, Daniels DL, Williams AL, Lynch R, Levine R (1986) A blinded clinical comparison of MR imaging and CT in neuroradiology. Radiology 160: 751–755

Hesselink JR, Healey ME, Press GA, Joseph PM, Goldberg HI, Bilaniuk LT (1988) Benefits of Gd-DTPA for MR imaging of intracranial abnormalities. JCAT 12: 266–274

Holland BA, Haas DK, Norman D, Brandt-Zawadzki M, Newton TH (1986) MRI of normal brain maturation. AJNR 7: 201–208

Holland BA, Kucharczyk W, Brandt-Zawadzki M, Norman D, Haas DA, Harper PS (1985) MR imaging of calcified intracranial lesions. Radiology 157: 353–356

Hubert DJ, Mueller E, Heubes P (1985) Oblique magnetic resonance imaging of normal structures. AJR 145: 843–846

Huynen CHJN, Ruijs JHJ, Tulleken CAF (1986) MRI of the brain and cervical spine: first choice in the detection of abnormalities. Diag Imag Clin Med 55: 61–65

Iio M, Yoshikawa K (1986) Textbook of brain spinal MRI diagnosis. Bunkodo, Tokyo (Japanese)

Kean DM, Worthington BS, Firth JL, Hawkes RC (1985) The effects of magnetic resonance imaging on different types of microsurgical clips. J Neurol Neurosurg Psychiat 48: 286–287

Kelly WM (1987) Image artifacts and technical limitations. In: Brant-Zawadzki M, Norman D (eds) Magnetic resonance imaging of the central nervous system. Raven Press, New York, pp43–82

Kilgore DP, Breger RK, Daniels DL, Pojunas KW, Williams AL, Haughton VM (1986) Cranial tissues: normal MR appearance after intravenous injection of Gd-DTPA. Radiology 160: 757–761

Kjos BO, Ehman RL, Brant-Zawadzki M, Kelly WM, Norman D, Newton TH (1985) Reproducibility of relaxation times and spin density calculated from MR imaging sequences: clinical study of the CNS. AJNR 6: 271–273

Koehler PR, Haughton VM, Daniels DL, Williams AL, Yetkin Z, Charles HC, Shutts D (1985) MR measurement of normal and pathologic brainstem diameters. AJNR 6: 425–427

Koenig H, Lenz M, Sauter R (1986) Temporal bone region: high resolution MR imaging using surface coils. Radiology 159: 191–194

Komiyama M, Yagura H, Baba M, Yasui T, Hakuba A, Nishimura S, Inoue Y (1987) MR imaging: possibility of tissue characterization of brain tumors using T_1 and T_2 values. AJNR 8: 65–70

Krol G, Galicich J, Arbit E, Sze G, Amster J (1988) Preoperative localization of intracranial lesions on MR. AJNR 9: 513–516

Kucharczyk W, Brant-Zawadzki M, Lemme-Plaghos L, Uske A, Kjos B, Feinberg DA, Norman D (1985) MR technology: effect of even-echo rephasing on calculated T2 values and T2 images. Radiology 157: 95–101

Kucharczyk W, Crawley AP, Kelly WM, Henkelman RM (1988) Effect of multislice interference on image contrast in T_2- and T_1-weighted MR images. AJNR 9: 443–451

Kucharczyk W, Kelly WM, Davis DO, Norman D, Newton TH (1986) Intracranial lesions: flow-related enhancement on MR images using time-of-flight effects. Radiology 161: 767–772

Kurauchi M, Murata T, Ezumi Y (1988) MRI contrast medium. Journal of Medical Imagings 8: 450–453 (Japanese)

LeBihan D, Breton E, Lallemand D, Grenier P, Cabanis E, Laval-Jeantet M (1986) MR imaging of intravoxel incoherent motions: applications to diffusion and perfusion in neurologic disorders. Radiology 161: 401–407

Leksell L, Herner T, Leksell D, Persson B, Lindquist C (1985) Visualisation of stereotactic radiolesions by nuclear magnetic resonance. J Neurol Neurosurg Psychiat 48: 19–20

Leksell L, Leksell D, Schwebel J (1985) Stereotaxis and nuclear magnetic resonance. J Neurol Neurosurg Psychiat 40: 14–18

Lewis CE, Prato FS, Drost DJ, Nicholson RL (1986) Comparison of respiratory triggering and gating techniques for the removal of respiratory artifacts in MR imaging. Radiology 160: 803–810

Ludeke KM, Roschmann P, Tischler R (1985) Susceptibility artifacts in NMR imaging. Magn Reson Imaging 3: 329–343

Lufkin RG, Pusey E, Stark DD, Brown R, Leikind B, Hanafee WN (1986) Boundary artifacts due to truncation errors in MR imaging. AJR 147: 1283–1287

Lunsford LD, Martinez AJ, Latchaw RE (1986) Stereotaxic surgery with a magnetic resonance and computerized tomography-compatible system. J Neurosurg 64: 872–878

MacDonald HL, Bell BA, Smith BA, Smith MA, Kean DM, Tocher JL, Douglas RH, Miller JD, Best JJ (1986) Correlation of human NMR T_1 values measured in vivo and brain water content. Br J Radiol 59: 355–357

Mamourian AC, Briggs RW (1986) Appearance of Pantopaque on MR images. Radiology 158: 457–460

Mamourian AC, Rhodes RE, Duda JJ, Towfighi J, White WS, Page RB, Cunningham DE, Lehman RA (1988) MR-directed brain biopsy: feasibility study. AJNR 9: 510–512

McNamara MT (1987) Paramagnetic contrast media for magnetic resonance imaging of the central nervous system. In: Brant-Zawadzki M, Norman D (eds) Magnetic resonance imaging of the central nervous system. Raven Press, New York, pp97–106

Mills TC, Ortendahl DA, Hylton NM, Crooks LE, Carlson JW, Kaufman L (1987) Partial flip angle MR imaging. Radiology 162: 531–539

Moseley IF (1986) Diagnostic imaging in neurological disease. Churchill Livingstone. Edinburgh

Norman D (1987) Vascular disease: hemorrhage. In: Brant-Zawadzki M, Norman D (eds) Magnetic resonance imaging of the central nervous system. Raven Press, New York, pp221–234

Oot RF, New PFJ, Pile-Spellman J, Rosen BR, Shoukimas GM, Davis KR (1986) The detection of intracranial calcification by MR. AJNR 7: 801–809

Perman WH, Moran PR, Moran RA, Bernstein MA (1986) Artifacts from pulsatile flow in MR imaging. JCAT 10: 473–483

Perman WH, Turski PA, Houston LW, Glover GH, Hayes CE (1986) Methodology of in vivo human sodium MR imaging at 1.5 T. Radiology 160: 811–820

Quencer RM, Hinks RS, Pattany PH, Horen M, Post MJD (1988) Improved MR imaging of the brain by using compensating gradients to suppress motion-induced artifacts. AJNR 9: 431–438

Roschmann P, Tischler R (1986) Surface coil proton MR imaging at 2T. Radiology 161: 251–255

Schenck JF, Foster TH, Henkes JL, Adams WJ, Hayes C, Hart HR Jr, Edelstein WA, Bottomley PA, Wehrli FW (1985) High-field surface coil MR imaging of localized anatomy. AJNR 6: 181–186

Schick RM, Wismer GL, Davis KR (1988) Magnetic susceptibility effects secondary to out-of-plane air in fast MR scanning. 9: 439–442

Schmiedl U, Ogan M, Paajamen H, Marotti M, Crooks LE, Brito AC, Brash RC (1987) Albumin labeled with Gd-DTPA as an intravascular, blood pool-enhancing agent for MR imaging: biodistribution and imaging studies. Radiology 162: 205–210

Shaw D (1987) Principles, methodology and applications of biomedical magnetic resonance. In: Wehrli FW, Shaw D, Kneeland B (eds) Chapter 1. VCH Publishers, New York

Shellock FG, Crues JV (1987) Temperature, heart rate, and blood pressure changes associated with clinical MR imaging at 1.5T. Radiology 163: 259–262

Sherman JL, Citrin CM (1986) Magnetic resonance demonstration of normal CSF flow. AJNR 7: 3–6

Sherman JL, Citrin CM, Gangarosa RE, Bowen BJ (1986) The MR of CSF pulsations in the spinal canal. AJNR 7: 879–884

Soulen RL, Budinger TF, Higgins CB (1985) Magnetic resonance imaging of prosthetic heart valves. Radiology 154: 705–707

Stack JP, Antoun NM, Jenkins JPR, Metcalfe R, Isherwood I. (1988) Gadolinium-DTPA as a contrast agent in magnetic resonance imaging of the brain. Neuroradiology 30: 145–154

Stark DD, Bradley WG (eds) (1988) Magnetic resonance imaging. Mosby, Saint Louis

Sze G, De Armond SJ, Brant-Zawadzki M, Davis RL, Norman D, Newton TH (1986) Foci of MRI signal (pseudolesions) anterior to the frontal horns: histologic correlations of a normal finding. AJR 147: 331–337

Takemoto K, Inoue Y, Hashimoto H, Shyakudo M, Matsumura Y, Nemoto Y, Fukuda T, Onoyama T, Hakuba A, Yagura H, Baba M (1985) Clinical experience of Gadolinium-DTPA: contrast enhanced MR imaging. Jpn J Clin Radiol 31:795–801 (English abstract)

Thomas DGT, Davis CH, Ingram S, Olney JS, Bydder GM, Young IR (1986) Stereotaxic biopsy of the brain under MR imaging control. AJNR 7: 161–163

Tsurada JS, Bradley WG (1987) MR detection of intracranial calcification: a phantom study. AJNR 8: 1049–1055

von Schulthess GK, Higgings CB (1985) Blood flow imaging with MR: spinphase phenomena. Radiology 157: 687–695

Walker MF, Souza SP, Dumoulin CL (1988) Quantitative flow measurement in phase contrast MR angiography. JCAT 12: 304–313

Wiener SN, Pzeszotarski MS, Droege RT, Pearlstein AE, Shafron M (1985) Measurement of pituitary gland height with MR imaging. AJNR 6: 717–722

Wismer GL, Buxton RB, Rosen BR, Fisel CR, Oot RF, Brady TJ, Davis KR (1988) Susceptibility induced MR line broadening: applications to brain iron mapping. JCAT 12: 259–265

Wolf GL, Joseph PM, Goldstein EJ (1987) Optimal pulsing sequences for MR contrast agents. AJR 147: 367–371

Yoshikawa K (1987) Sufficient knowledge of MRI, necessary for neurosurgeons. Neurological Surgery 15: 365–372 (English abstract)

Young IR, Khenia S, Thomas DGT, Davis CH, Gadian DG, Cox IJ, Ross BD, Bydder GM (1987) Clinical magnetic susceptibility mapping of the brain. JCAT 11: 2–6

Zimmerman RA, Bilaniuk LT, Johnson MG, Hershey B, Jaffe S, Gomori JM, Goldberg HI, Grossman RI (1986) MRI of central nervous system: early clinical results. AJNR 7: 587–594

Zimmerman RD, Fleming CA, Lee BCP, Saint-Louis LA, Deck MDF (1986) Periventricular hyperintensity as seen by magnetic resonance: prevalence and significance. AJNR 7: 13–20

MRI of the CNS
Disorders

6 Intracranial Tumors

The accuracy of radiological diagnosis of brain tumors has improved remarkably with the introduction of MRI. The resolution of MRI had been considered poorer than that of CT; but with the introduction of the superconductive MRI and the development of gadolinium diethylenetriamine pentaacetic acid (Gd-DTPA), the quality of MRI as well as its accuracy in diagnosis have far surpassed those of CT. This has now often rendered the use of CT unnecessary.

Tumor detectability by MRI is far superior to that by CT, and the anatomical relationship of the tumor to the surrounding tissues is also much easier to comprehend. In an MRI diagnosis of brain tumors, principally the T_1 and T_2 weighted SE images are used. In many brain tumors, both T_1 and T_2 are prolonged, and although the signal intensity is low in the T_1 weighted image it is usually high on the T_2 weighting. The subtle differences in the T_1 and T_2 images among the different tumors are important tools in differential diagnosis. In other words, even though tumors possess similar characteristics, they can be differentiated on T_1 and T_2 weighting.

There are still difficulties to overcome. However, because of the relationship between tumor tissue and its metabolism, it is possible to investigate the nature of tumors from their concentration of minerals such as sodium, phosphorus, etc. At present, although it is used for differential diagnosis, MRI does not always clarify the biological characteristics of tumors. Furthermore, the differential diagnosis of gliomas and radiation necroses is still problematic. One of the shortcomings of MRI is its inadequacy in the detection of calcifications.

These problems will be alleviated to some extent with the introduction of Gd-DTPA, which enhances tumor image due to the shortening of T_1 and T_2 intervals, thereby contributing to the establishment of the diagnosis. Tumor tissue is enhanced in about 8 min after intravenous injection of Gd-DTPA, but enhancement of necrotic tissue within the tumor occurs more slowly, becoming maximal in about 1 hour. If the regions without blood-brain barrier (e.g. hypothalamus, pituitary stalk, pituitary gland, pineal body, choroid plexus, and area postrema) are excluded, normal brain tissue is mostly nonenhancing. Perifocal edema of cerebral tumors is rarely delineated and detecting the presence of tumor infiltration still needs further study. Gd-DTPA provides remarkable enhancement of images, especially in benign tumors, and there is clear enhancement of lesions such as acoustic neurinomas and meningiomas in the T_1 weighted image. However, other tumors such as pituitary adenomas, hamartomas, and choristomas are mostly either unaffected or are only slightly enhanced.

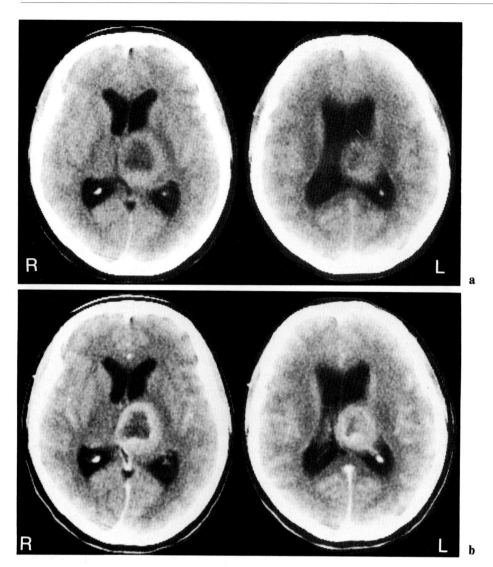

Fig. 6.1. Glioblastoma. A 34-year-old female. The patient had started having headaches and vomiting about 1 month prior to consultation. The vomiting was frequent, profuse, and usually occurred following meals. She was referred to our clinic on a suspicion of intracranial pathology by her general physician. Upon admission, an examination revealed the presence of psychiatric symptoms and Parinaud's sign.

a, b *CT scan.* A round isodensity mass is seen in the left thalamus on plain CT. The inner portion is seen as a low density, with the mass extending into the lateral ventricle. On the enhanced CT scan, the mass displays the characteristic ring-enhancement.

c *Angiography.* Vertebral angiography shows stretching and posterior displacement of the lateral posterior choroidal artery. The tumor stain is seen in the capillary and venous phases.

d–f *MRI.* The tumor is seen as a low signal intensity in the T_1 weighted image and as a high signal intensity in the T_2 weighted image. No peritumoral edema is present. Biopsy was performed through a parieto-occipital approach, and pathological study of the tumor returned a diagnosis of glioblastoma.

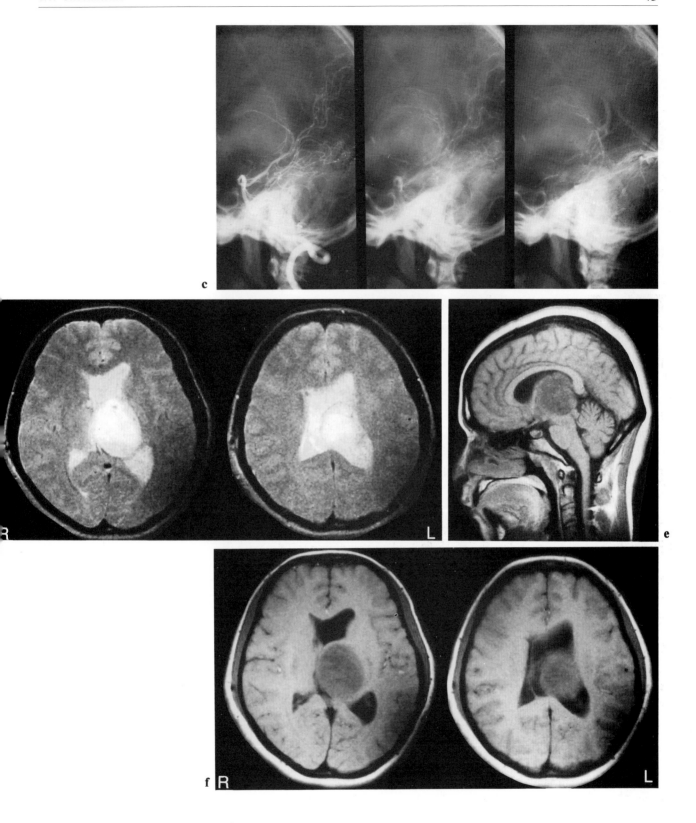

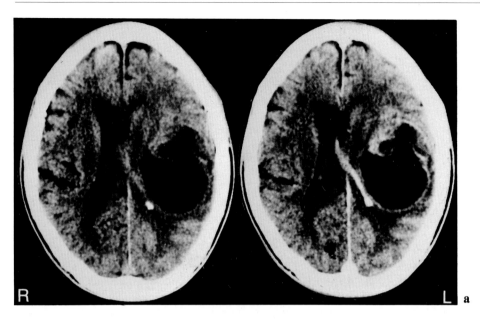

Fig. 6.2. Glioblastoma. A 78-year-old male. The onset of clumsiness and forgetfulness was insidious and revealed by the patient's upsetting bowls while eating and mixing up the names of his children. The condition gradually worsened and culminated in a convulsive seizure on the morning he was brought to our clinic. The physical examination upon arrival revealed the presence of Gerstmann's syndrome, right hemiparesis, exaggerated deep tendon reflexes, and the presence of pathological reflexes.

a *CT scan.* In the plain axial CT scan, a round low density area is seen extending from the left temporal to the parietal regions with marked mass effect. The ventricles are compressed and there is midline shift. The mass is enhanced in a ring-like fashion and its anterior portion is enhanced in the manner of mural nodule.

b, c *MRI.* In the T$_1$ weighted axial image, a low intensity mass is present from the left temporal to the parietal regions — findings which are consistent with those of CT. The mass appears as an area of slightly higher intensity than CSF. Perifocal edema anterior and posterior to the mass also appears as high intensity. In the coronal and sagittal images enhanced by Gd-DTPA, the mass is enhanced in a ring-like fashion. The mural nodule-like portion in the CT scan is markedly enhanced. The mass was histologically diagnosed as a glioblastoma.

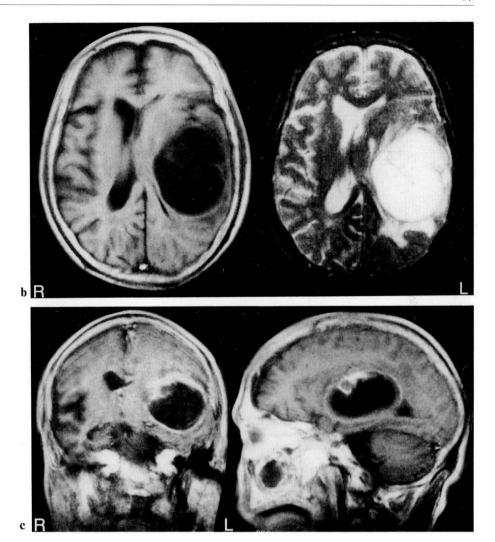

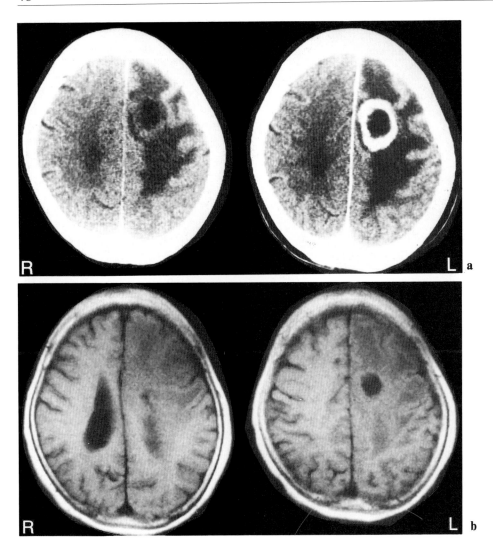

Fig. 6.3. Glioblastoma. A 76-year-old female. The onset of a gradually worsening right hemiparesis occurred about 1 month prior to our being consulted. On admission, the right hemiparesis was the only significant neurological finding.

a *CT scan.* A ring-enhanced mass with diffuse perifocal edema is seen in the left frontal lobe.

b–d *MRI.* The tumor is seen as a low signal intensity in the T_1 weighted image but as a high signal intensity on T_2 weighting. The extent of perifocal edema is well demonstrated on T_2. Biopsy was performed through a left frontal transcortical approach, and the tumor was diagnosed on pathological study as a glioblastoma.

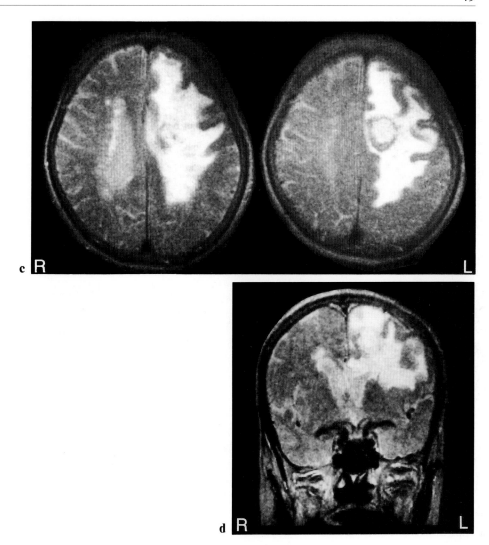

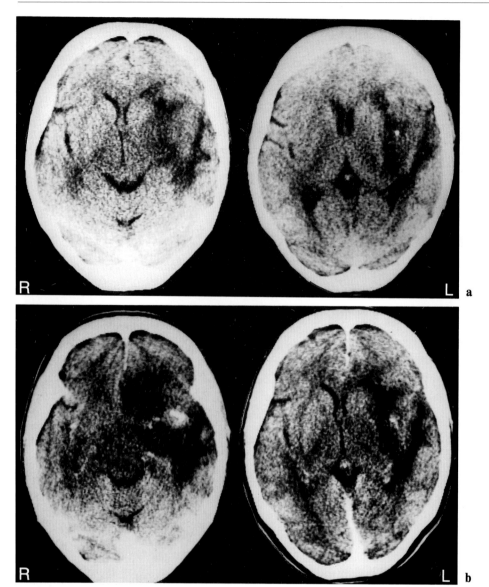

Fig. 6.4. Astrocytoma. A 49-year-old female. The patient reported having had strange floating sensations since approximately 1 year prior to visiting our clinic. This had gradually become worse and was often accompanied by episodes of falling. Physical examination revealed no obvious neurological abnormalities.

a, b *CT scan.* The plain CT scan shows a low density area in the left temporal lobe. There is a slight mass effect which is partially enhanced by an injection of contrast medium.

c, d *MRI.* In comparison with the surrounding brain, the low density area in the left temporal lobe of CT is seen as a low signal intensity in the T_1 weighted image and as a high signal intensity in the T_2 image. There is a slight mass effect but the boundary between mass and edema is not clearly demarcated. There is no evidence of intratumoral hemorrhage. The mass was found to be an astrocytoma grade 2 upon pathological examination of the biopsy. In gliomas, both T_1 and T_2 are markedly prolonged in the tumors and edema making their differentiation difficult. To overcome this problem, it might be useful to intensify the image with Gd-DTPA.

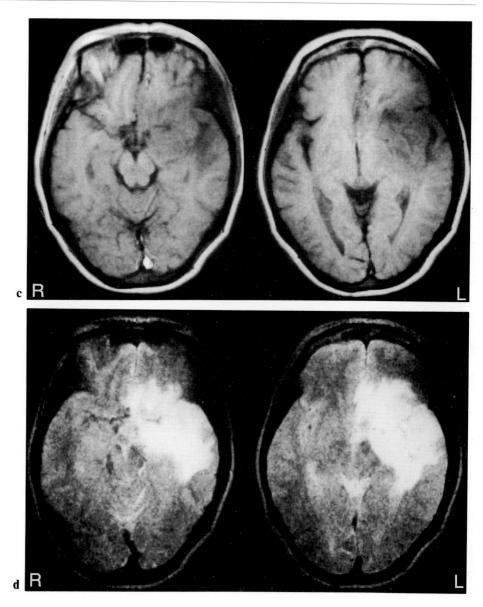

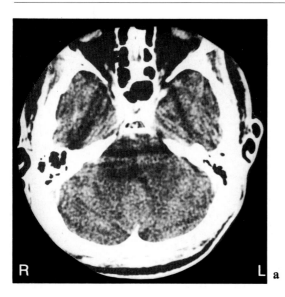

Fig. 6.5. Pontine Glioma. A 32-year-old male. The patient came to our clinic with a history of double-vision and gradually worsening left hemiparesis that had started a few months previously. A neurological examination revealed a right oculomotor paresis, abducens palsy, a right facial weakness, and a left hemiparesis with exaggerated deep tendon reflexes.

a *CT scan.* A low density mass is seen to the right of the midline in the pons in the contrast-enhanced scan. The fourth ventricle is shifted in the opposite direction with moderate mass effect.

b, c *MRI.* A lesion is seen in an area corresponding to that of the CT scan. It appears as a low intensity in the T_1 weighted image, but as a high intensity in the T_2 weighted image. In the T_1 weighted sagittal image, a well-circumscribed low intensity mass is observed in the center of the lower pons. The fourth ventricle is displaced to the left side and is shown as a low intensity in the T_1 weighted image and a slightly high intensity on the T_2 weighting. The mass, which was vague in the CT scan, is clearly demonstrated in both the T_1 and T_2 weighted images. Because there is no perifocal edema, the tumor is clearly demarcated. A surgical specimen taken at operation was diagnosed as a low-grade astrocytoma.

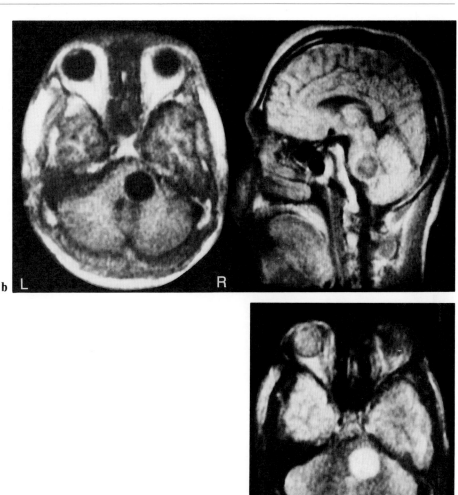

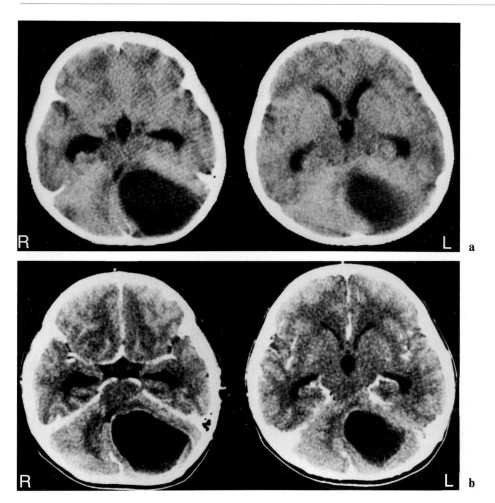

Fig. 6.6. Cystic Cerebellar Astrocytoma. A 4-year-old male. The child was delivered spontaneously following a normal full-term pregnancy. At 18 months of age, he was noted to have speech retardation and was taken to a pediatrician who noted a tumor on the CT scan and referred him to our clinic.

a, b *CT scan.* The entire area of the left cerebellar hemisphere is occupied by a large cystic mass. Part of the cyst wall is enhanced following an injection of contrast medium, although there is no apparent mural nodule. The fourth ventricle is displaced and deformed, and hydrocephalus is present.

c–f *MRI.* The cyst wall is demonstrated as a low signal intensity in the T_1 weighted image and as a high intensity in the T_2 weighted image. There is also prolongation of both the T_1 and T_2 values. The sagittal image shows narrowing of the fourth ventricle and aqueduct, and downward displacement of the cerebellar tonsils. The cyst was opened and its wall was biopsied. The tumor was diagnosed on pathological examination as an astrocytoma grade 2.

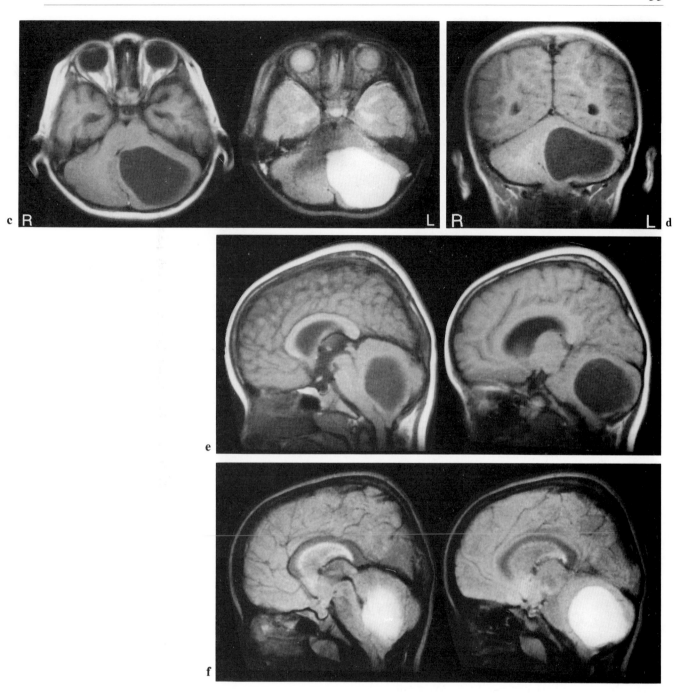

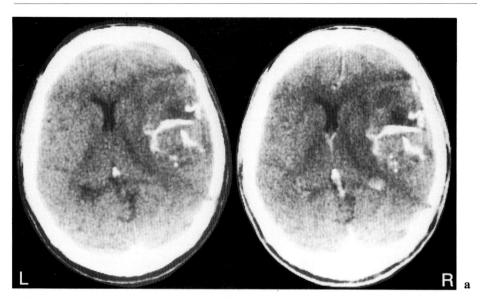

Fig. 6.7. Oligodendroglioma. A 40-year-old male. The patient had consulted a physician because of seizure attacks 7 years ago. A CT scan done at the time revealed what was suspected to be a brain tumor in the right frontoparietal region. This was partially removed at another hospital and the histological diagnosis was that of an oligodendroglioma. He developed heaviness of the head and left hemiparesis a few months prior to our examination. The CT scan revealed what was believed to be a recurrence of the tumor and the patient was subsequently referred to our clinic.

a *CT scan.* In the axial section of plain CT, an iso to slightly high density mass with a ring-shaped high density suggesting calcification is seen in the right frontoparietal region. High density spots also appear within the mass. There is shift of the midline structures with ventricular compression. The image of the mass is slightly enhanced following injection of contrast medium.

b–e *MRI.* In the T_1 coronal image, an iso to slightly high intensity mass is seen extending from the parietal region to the Sylvian fissure; low intensity spots (or areas believed to represent calcifications) are visible within it. The lesion is located in the motor and sensory areas and extends medially into the operculum and external capsule. In the T_2 weighted image the mass is seen as inhomogeneous, i.e., of a markedly high intensity. Branches of the middle cerebral artery are shown as markedly low intensity spots due to the absence of signal (signal void), and calcifications are of relatively low intensity. Perifocal edema may be included in the high intensity, which would be difficult to differentiate from tumor. In the T_1 weighted sagittal image, an iso to slightly high intensity mass is seen in the right frontoparietal region. It extends to the Sylvian fissure and partially infiltrates into the superior temporal gyrus. There are scattered low intensity areas representing calcification within the tumor. In the T_2 weighted image, the tumor is shown as an inhomogeneous low intensity with a slight low intensity due to calcification, and as a markedly low intensity of the middle cerebral artery.

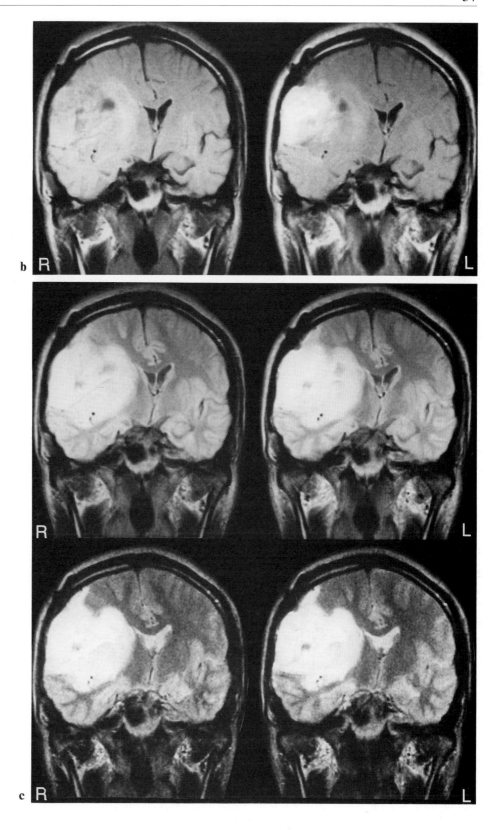

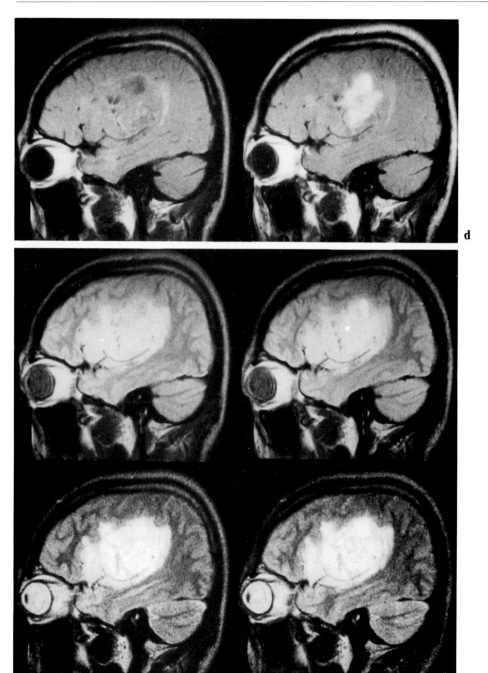

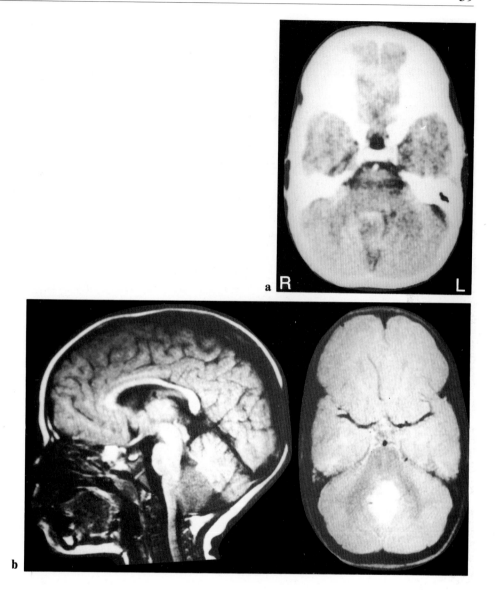

Fig. 6.8. Fourth Ventricle Ependymoma. A 3-year-old female. The child was delivered normally following a full-term and uneventful pregnancy. She started having episodes of vomiting and disturbances of gait for about 1 month with increasing frequency. The first medical examination revealed papilledema, a broad-based gait, and positive Romberg's signs, and she was referred to our clinic for further evaluation.

a *CT scan.* A poorly defined slightly high density mass is seen in the midline; the fourth ventricle is deformed and pushed anterolaterally. There is no hydrocephalus.

b *MRI.* A slightly low signal intensity mass is seen in the fourth ventricle, extending down to the foramen magnum and appearing to infiltrate into the medulla oblongata. The tumor was removed via a suboccipital craniectomy and histologically diagnosed as an ependymoma.

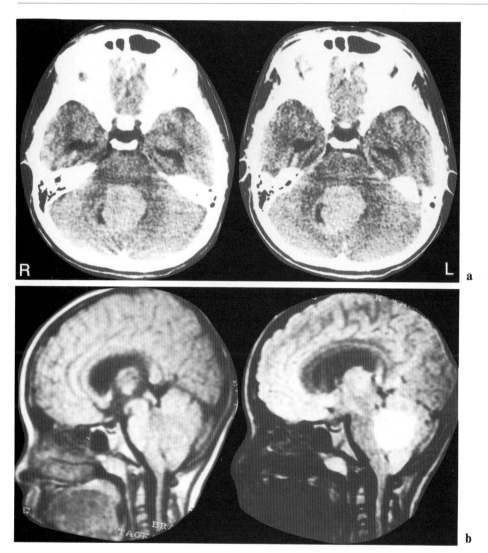

Fig. 6.9. Medulloblastoma. A 6-year-old female. The child developed gradually worsening headaches followed by nausea about 1 month prior to a medical examination. A CT scan revealed a brain tumor and the patient was referred to our clinic. A neurological examination upon admission revealed right cerebellar signs and an ataxic gait.

a *CT scan.* The image of a high density mass intensified by injection of a contrast medium is seen in the vermis. There is also mild ventricular dilatation.

b *MRI.* The tumor appears as a low signal intensity area in the T_1 weighted image. It is particularly well demonstrated in the sagittal section. The tumor was removed though a posterior fossa craniectomy, and histological examination confirmed it to be a medulloblastoma.

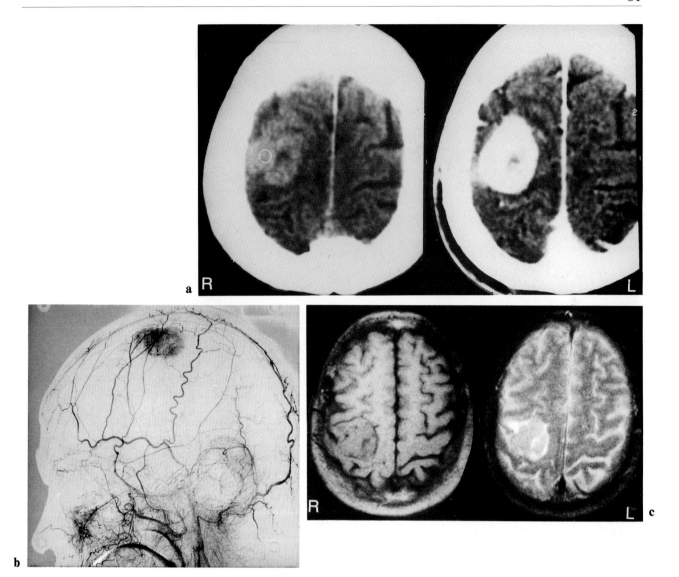

Fig. 6.10. Convexity Meningioma. A 61-year-old male. The patient presented with a 5 month history of numbness of the fingers and weakness of the muscles of the left hand.

a *CT scan.* A slightly high density mass is seen in the right parietal region on the plain CT scan which is markedly enhanced by injection of contrast medium. No peritumoral edema is present.

b *Angiography.* A right external carotid angiography shows a tumor stain which is supplied by the middle meningeal, superficial temporal, and occipital arteries.

c *MRI.* In both the T_1 and T_2 weighted images, the mass is shown as an area of isointensity. There is a peritumoral band between the mass and surrounding tissues suggesting that it is an extra-axial mass. In many cases of meningiomas, the tumor is of isointensity in both the T_1 and T_2 images. In about 10% of the cases, however, it may be seen as a low intensity in the T_1 weighted image and a high signal intensity in the T_2 weighted image. Meningiomas often exhibit peritumoral bands and venous capsules in which a low signal band surrounds the tumor (caused by tumor vessels) in the T_2 weighted image. In parasagittal meningiomas, the coronal image is useful in demonstrating obstruction of the superior sagittal sinus.

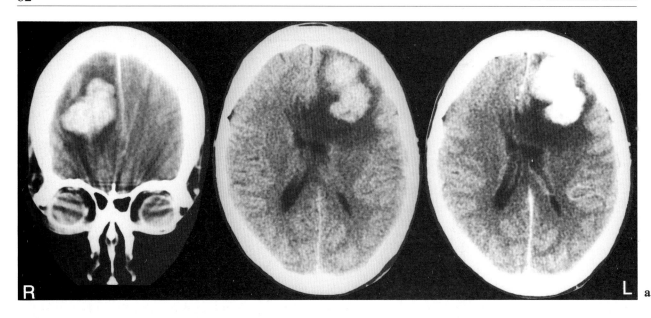

Fig. 6.11. Meningioma. A 44-year-old female. The patient consulted a physician following a head injury (type 2). A CT scan which was performed to rule out intracranial involvement revealed a brain tumor, and the patient was referred to our clinic. The neurological examination was unremarkable except for a slight hemiparesis.

a *CT scan.* A homogeneously enhanced mass with perifocal edema is seen in the left frontal region.

b, c *MRI.* The tumor is shown as an isointensity in the T_1 and T_2 weighted images, and is markedly enhanced with Gd-DTPA. Perifocal edema is shown as a low intensity in the T_1 weighted image and as a high intensity in the T_2 weighted image. The tumor was removed through a left frontal craniotomy and histological examination diagnosed the lesion to be a meningotheliomatous meningioma.

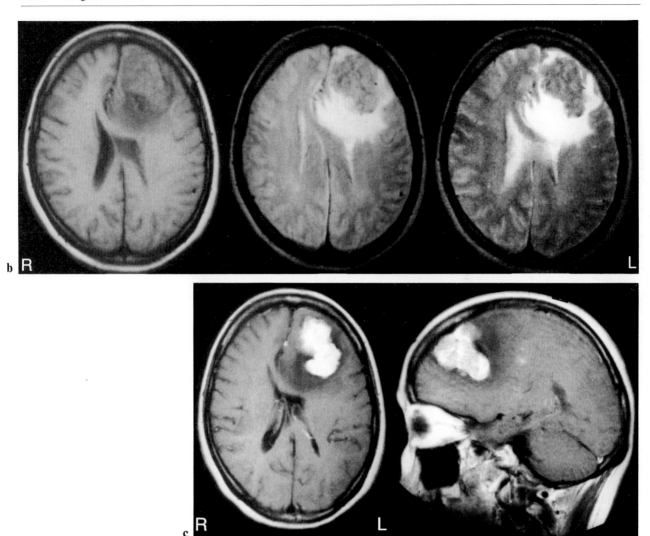

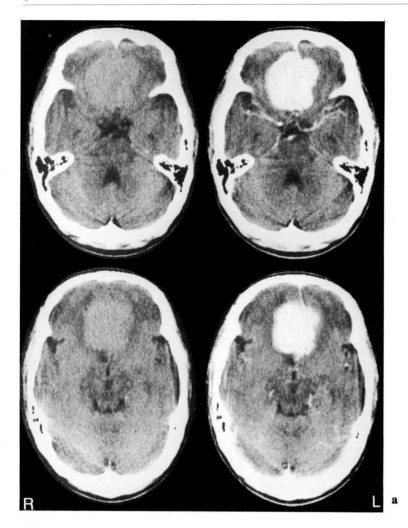

R L **a**

Fig. 6.12. Olfactory Groove Meningioma. A 36-year-old male. The patient had first had a convulsive seizure 4 years ago, followed by frequent attacks for which he consulted a physician. A CT scan was done revealing a brain tumor and the patient was referred to our clinic. A neurological examination revealed left anosmia, left optic atrophy and a right papilledema.

a *CT scan.* In the plain axial CT, a slightly high density mass is seen in the midline of the anterior cranial fossa. The image is homogeneously enhanced following injection of a contrast medium.

b–e *Angiogram.* On right carotid angiograms, frontopolar and pericallosal branches of the anterior cerebral artery are displaced upward (**b,c**), and a tumor stain (**d,e**) fed by anterior and posterior ethmoidal arteries is seen in the capillary to venous phase.

f–h *MRI.* In the axial T$_1$ weighted image, an iso to low density well circumscribed mass appears in the midline of the anterior cranial fossa (as in the CT scan). In the T$_2$ weighted image, the mass is shown as a homogeneously high intensity and has a peritumoral band within the normal brain material suggesting an extra-axial mass. Low intensity spots within the tumor suggest calcifications. The image is enhanced with an injection of Gd-DTPA. Total removal of the mass was effected through a bifrontal craniotomy, and histological examination returned a diagnosis of meningotheliomatous meningioma.

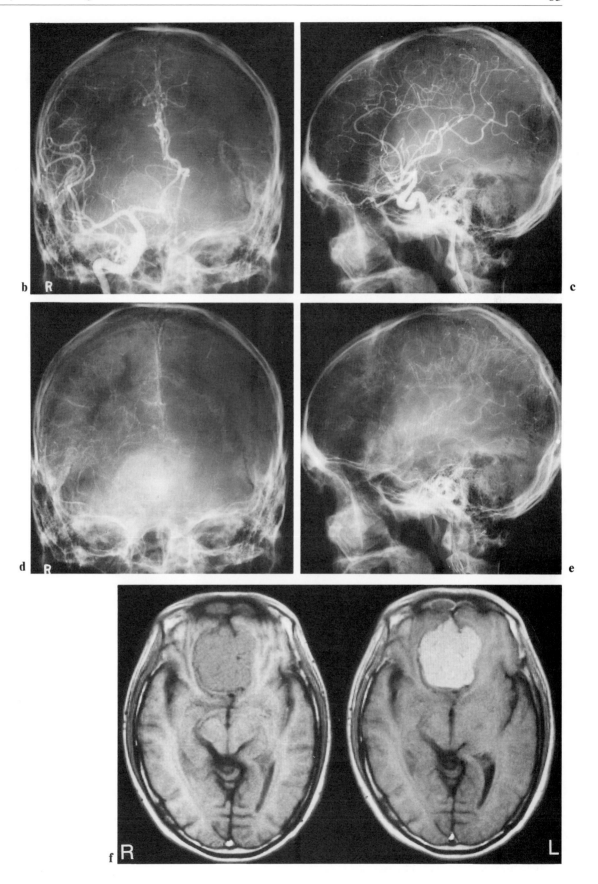

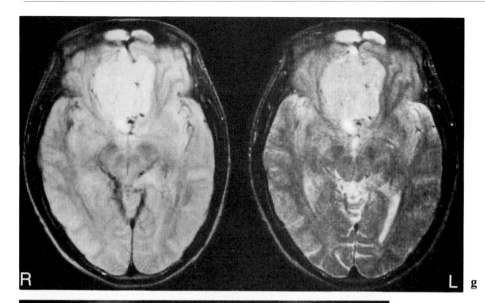

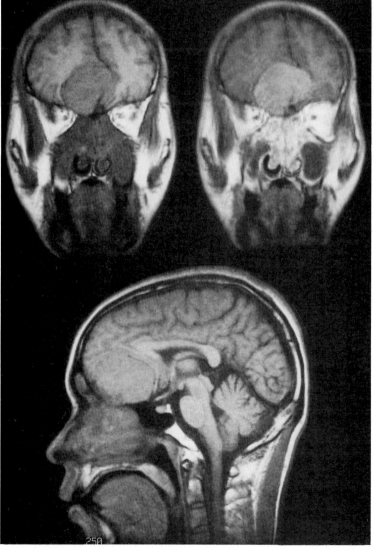

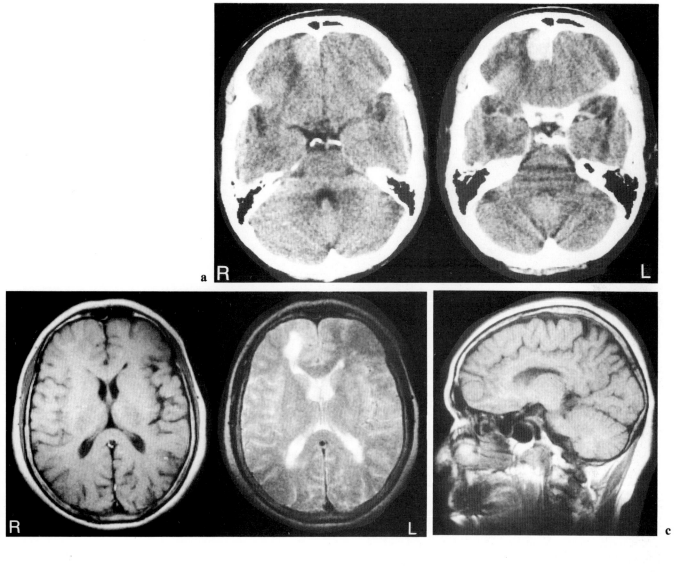

Fig. 6.13. Falx Meningioma. A 61-year-old female. The patient consulted us because of headaches and poor vision of the right eye which had started about 1 month ago. A physical examination confirmed papilledema of the right eye.

a *CT scan.* A slightly high density mass is present in the right frontal region. The image, which was homogeneously enhanced following the injection of a contrast medium, shows the mass to measure about 2 cm in diameter with no remarkable mass effect.

b, c *MRI.* The lesion is seen as an isointense area in both the T_1 and T_2 weighted images. Peritumoral edema is observed as a high signal intensity in the T_2 weighted image. In the sagittal image a band is seen in the interval between the tumor and the brain parenchyma, suggesting an extra-axial mass. The tumor was diagnosed as a falx meningioma based on the CT and MRI characteristics.

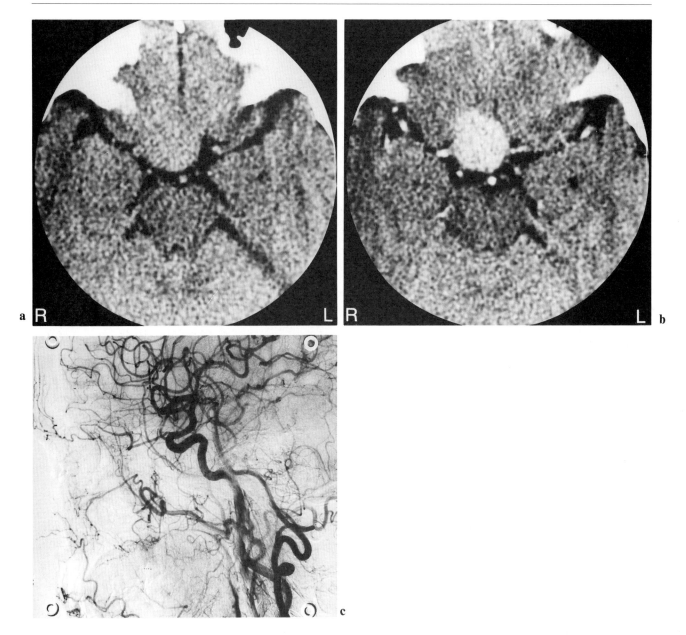

Fig. 6.14. Tuberculum Sellae Meningioma. A 60-year-old male. The patient presented to us with a 1 month history of headaches. A neurological examination revealed no remarkable findings.

a, b *CT scan.* A slightly high density mass is seen extending from the intrasellar to the suprasellar compartment. An injection of contrast medium produced homogeneous enhancement of the mass.

c *Angiography.* The carotid siphon is closed but there is no obvious tumor stain.

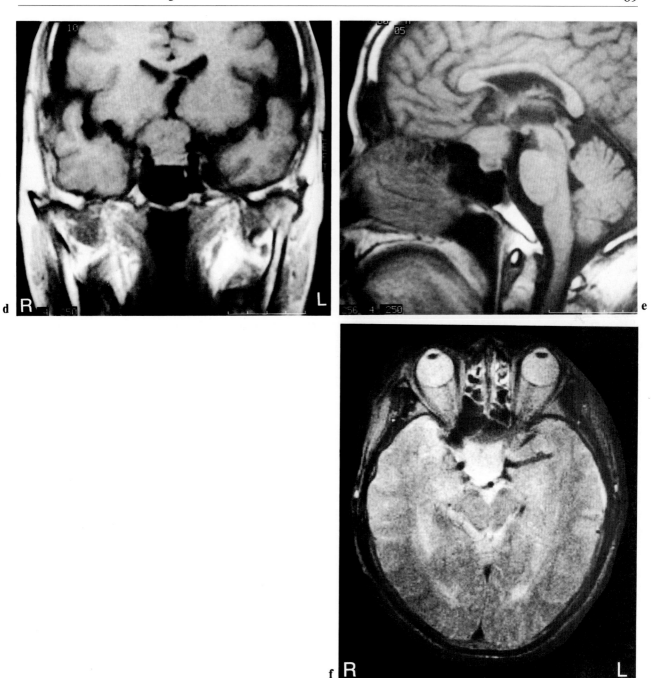

d–f *MRI*. An isointensity mass is present in the suprasellar region in the T₁ weighted image. The optic chiasm is pushed upwards from below and is flattened. In the T₂ weighted image, the mass shows an iso to slightly high signal intensity. From these findings and the fact that there was no ballooning of the sella, the mass was suspected to be a meningioma.

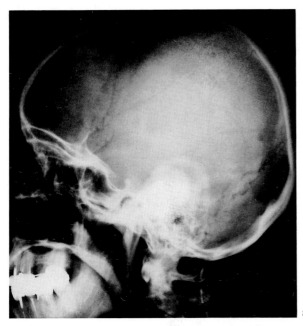

Fig. 6.15. Cerebellopontine Angle Meningioma. A 51-year-old female. The patient had noticed numbness in the right half of her face and tongue for about 1 year. A neurological examination revealed loss of the corneal reflex in the right eye, hyperesthesia of the right half of the face (V_1–V_3), decreased hearing acuity, and loss of the gag reflex on the right side.

a *Skull X-ray.* An elliptical calcification is seen in the right CP angle; the internal auditory meatuses are symmetrical.

b *CT scan.* A high density mass is seen in the right CP angle. It is well-circumscribed and is attached to the petrous bone. The fourth ventricle is slightly deformed.

c, d *MRI.* The tumor is shown as an isointense mass in both the T_1 and T_2 weighted images. The signal void observed in the posteromedial portion corresponds to calcification. Compression of the mass against the brainstem is well demonstrated in the coronal image. Following surgical excision of the mass, it was histologically verified as a psammomatous meningioma.

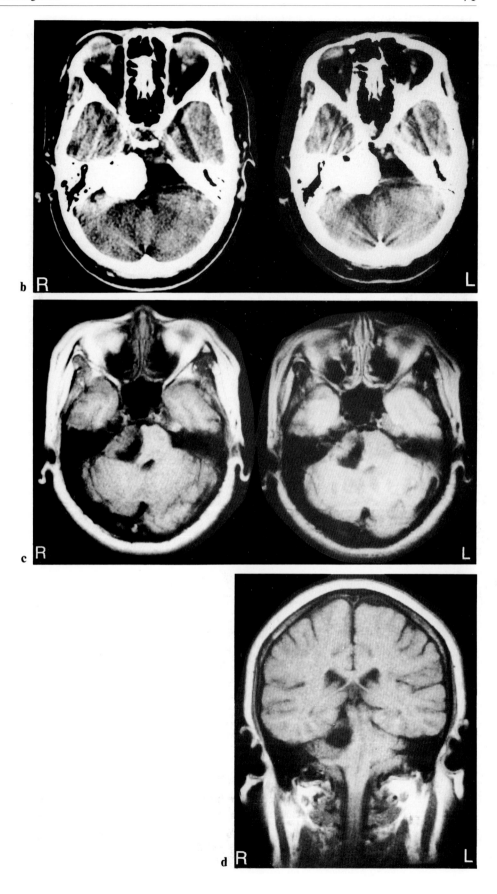

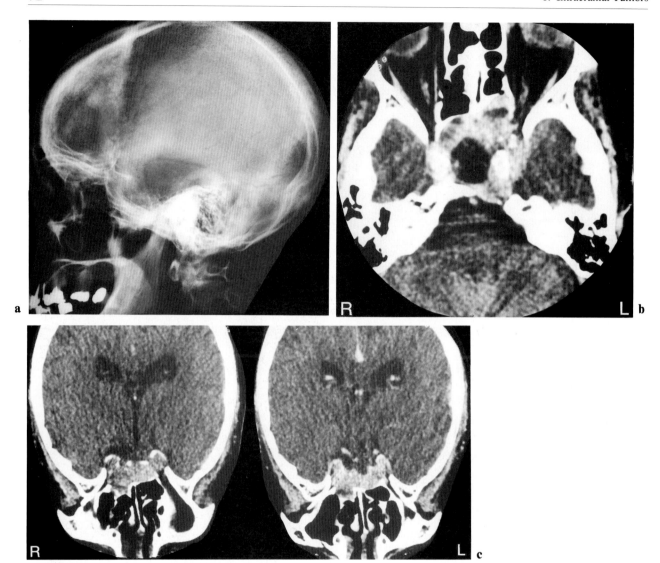

Fig. 6.16. Prolactinoma. A 65-year-old female. The patient developed amenorrhea at 30 years of age and was referred to our clinic because of galactorrhea. A hormonal examination had revealed plasma prolactin (PRL) elevated to 1500 ng/ml. There was no visual field defect and her visual acuity was normal.

a *Skull X-ray.* Plain skull films show an enlargement of the sella and decalcification of the anterior and posterior clinoid processes.

b, c *CT scan.* A slightly high density mass is seen in and around the sphenoid sinus and the image is homogeneously enhanced by an injection of a contrast medium.

d–g *MRI.* A tumor is seen extending from the sphenoid air sinus to the cavernous sinus. Invasion of the tumor around the internal carotid artery is well demonstrated in the sagittal image. There is no suprasellar extension and the sella is empty.

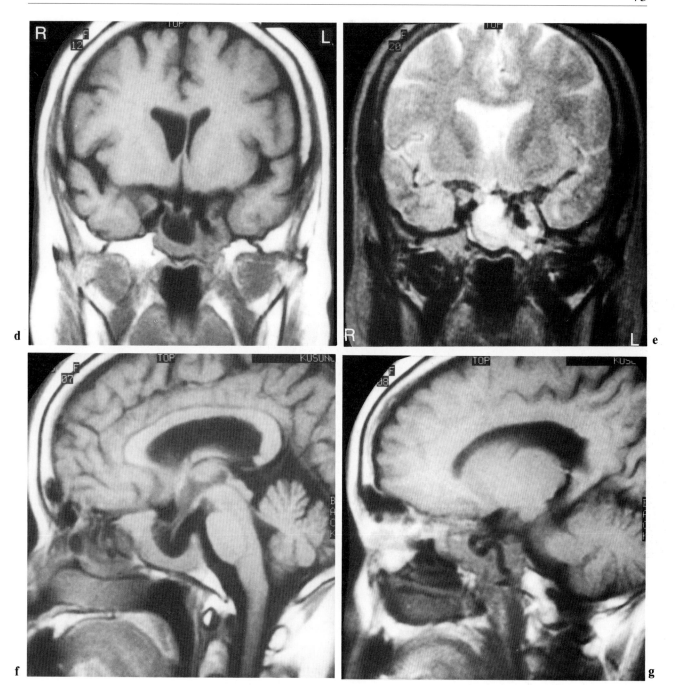

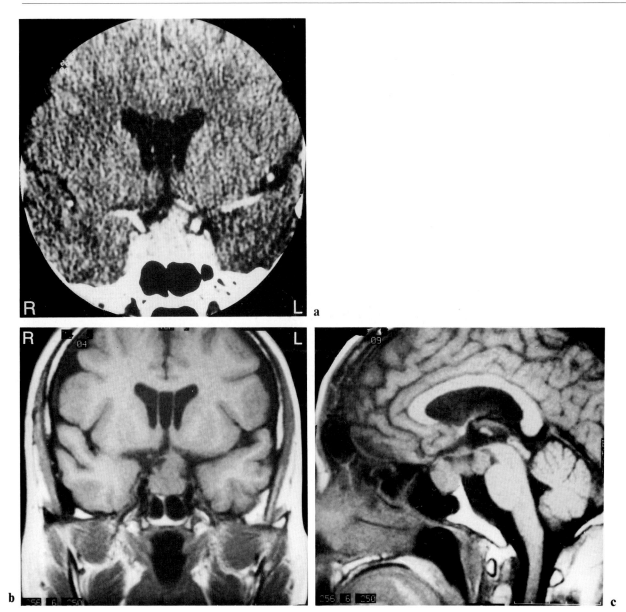

Fig. 6.17. Pituitary Adenoma. A 29-year-old male. The patient sought medical attention because of diminishing libido and easy fatigability. Serum prolactin (PRL) was found to be elevated to 458 ng/ml; he was referred to our clinic for further evaluation. The neurological examination was unremarkable.

a *CT scan.* A homogeneously enhanced mass is present in the intra- and suprasellar region. The A_1 portion of the anterior cerebral artery is elevated and cavum septi pellucidi is present.

b, c *MRI.* The tumor is shown as an isointensity mass extending upwards and to the left. The optic chiasm is slightly compressed from below and the tumor can be seen to extend immediately anteriorly to the midbrain in the sagittal image. Histological examination of the tumor identified a chromophobe adenoma. MRI is very useful in detecting pituitary adenomas. It efficiently displays numerous features including the degree of compression of the tumor against the optic chiasm, invasion into the cavernous sinus, shift in position of the pituitary stalk, and unilateral bulging of the pituitary gland.

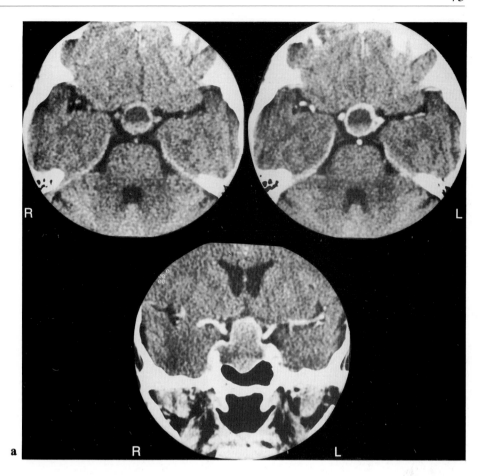

Fig. 6.18. Nonfunctioning Pituitary Adenoma. A 63-year-old female. The patient had earlier consulted an ophthalmologist with complaints of pain in the right eye and diplopia. A visual field defect and weakness of the right inferior oblique muscle were present, and a plain craniogram revealed a ballooned sella turcica. The patient was subsequently referred to our clinic. Endocrinological studies neither revealed diabetes insipidus nor any other abnormalities.

a *CT scan.* The plain axial CT scan indicates a round mass with a low density in the anterior half and a high density in the posterior half. Injection of a contrast medium produces ring-enhancement. In the coronal image, the mass shows a low density within a suprasellar extension from within the intrasellar compartment.

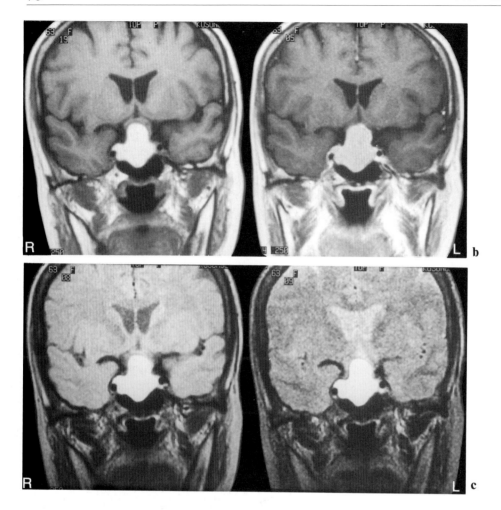

b–e *MRI*. In the coronal T_1 weighted image, the portion which appears as a slightly high to a low density in the CT scan is shown as a high signal intensity. The mass extends from the intrasellar compartment to the floor of the third ventricle. The images of the tumor capsule and tissue are markedly enhanced by Gd-DTPA in the floor of the ventricle. In the central part of the axial image, a fluid level is visible with a high intensity in the upper part and a low intensity in the lower part. The same findings are seen in the sagittal image. The lower layer may represent collections of sedimented blood or highly proteinaceous fluid. The tumor was removed through frontal craniotomy and diagnosed as a pituitary adenoma. The cyst content was a coffee-like fluid, and the pathology was considered to be pituitary apoplexy.

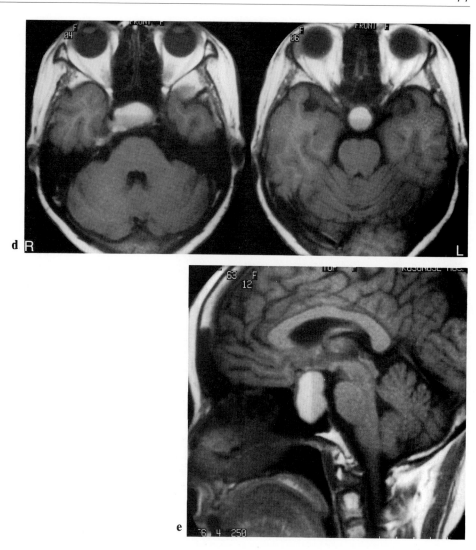

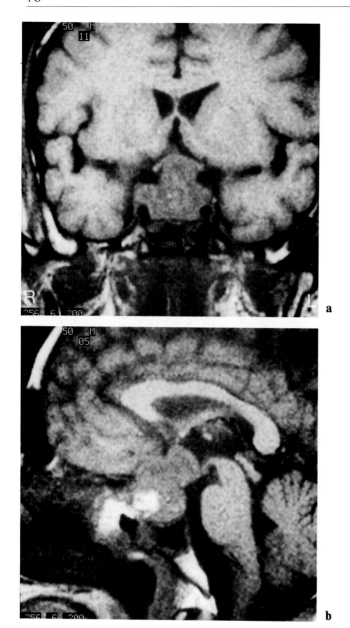

Fig. 6.19. Nonfunctioning Pituitary Adenoma (Postoperative status). A 50-year-old male. The patient underwent transsphenoidal surgery for a pituitary adenoma about 6 months before the present evaluation. The only significant neurological finding preoperatively was a bitemporal hemianopsia. MRI was performed during a follow-up examination.

a, b *MRI*. A large residual tumor is present in the intra- and suprasellar region. It compresses the optic chiasm from below and invades the cavernous sinuses on both sides. A high signal intensity area within the tumor represents fat which was packed into it during the previous surgery.

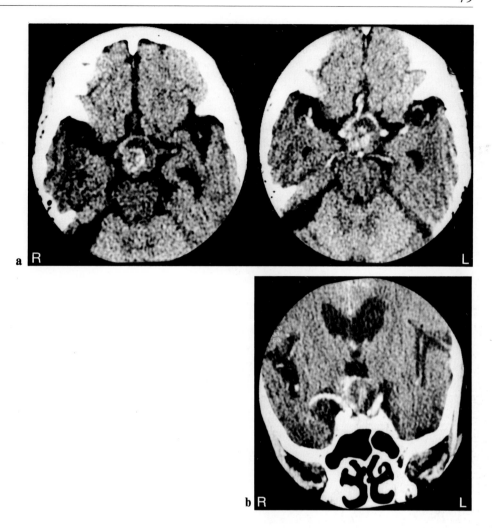

Fig. 6.20. Craniopharyngioma. A 78-year-old male. Frontal headaches appeared several months prior the patient's consulting our service. One month ago he had noticed a decrease in the visual acuity of his right eye. Past medical history included an episode of cerebral infarction three years previously. Neurological examination upon admission revealed a bitemporal hemianopsia and a right hemiparesis.

a, b *CT scan.* There is a calcified cystic mass in the suprasellar region. The image of the solid portion is enhanced following the injection of a contrast medium, but the cyst component remains unchanged. Extension of the tumor into the third ventricle is evident in the coronal scan.

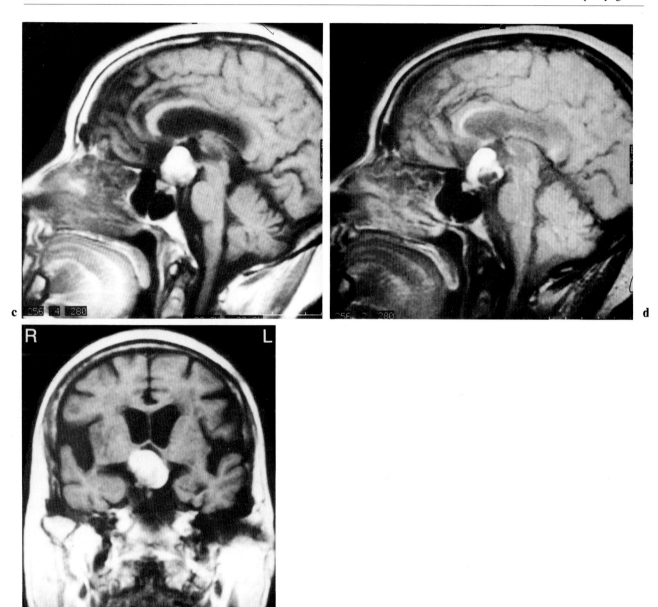

c–e *MRI*. A high signal intensity mass is seen in the suprasellar region in both the T_1 and T_2 weighted images. A high signal intensity area in the T_1 weighted image is considered to be due to the presence of cholesterin within the cyst. The coronal image shows compression of the optic chiasm from below. The mass can be differentiated from a pituitary adenoma since the normal pituitary gland can be observed in the sella. The calcified portion in the mass on CT corresponds to the signal void area.

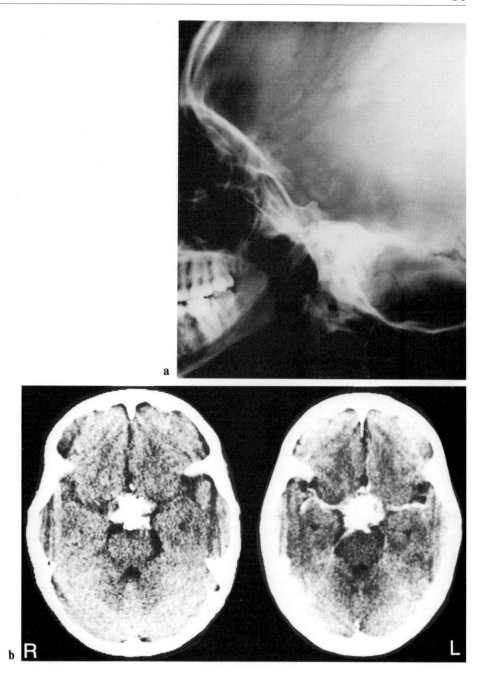

Fig. 6.21. Craniopharyngioma. A 25-year-old female. The patient was observed to be of somewhat short stature at 6 years of age when she started having frequent episodes of vomiting. A medical examination revealed a brain tumor but no operation was performed. Her visual acuity started to deteriorate around 14 years of age and she developed polyuria which gradually worsened. Upon admission into our hospital, a visual examination showed light perception in the right eye and complete blindness in the left eye. Fundoscopy revealed optic atrophy.

a *Skull X-ray.* There is a suprasellar calcification, decalcification of the dorsum sellae, and a saucer-like sella.

b *CT scan.* The suprasellar cistern is occupied by a calcified mass which is slightly enhanced by injection of contrast medium. There is no visible cyst.

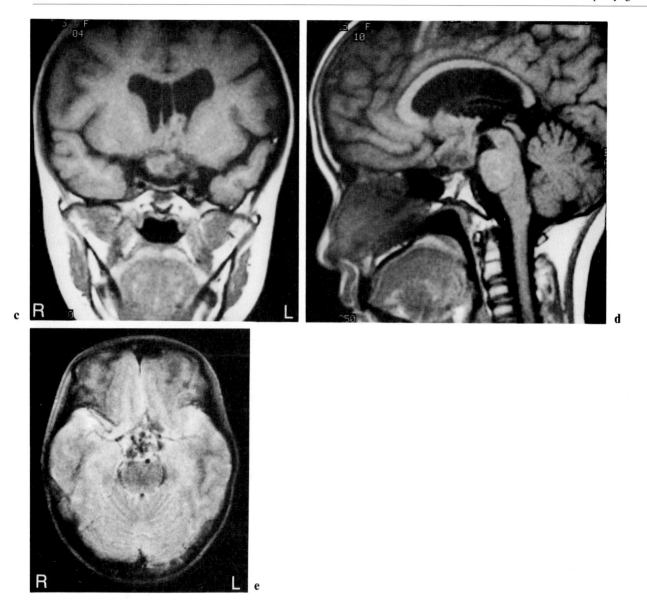

c–e *MRI*. There is a suprasellar mass with a postero superior extension. The tumor involves the optic chiasm and tract. In the T_1 and T_2 weighted images, the mass is seen as an isointensity area. The pituitary gland, which is depressed downward, can be seen in the sella in the sagittal image. The signal void area represents calcification seen in the T_2 weighted image. Cavum septi pellucidi is well demonstrated.

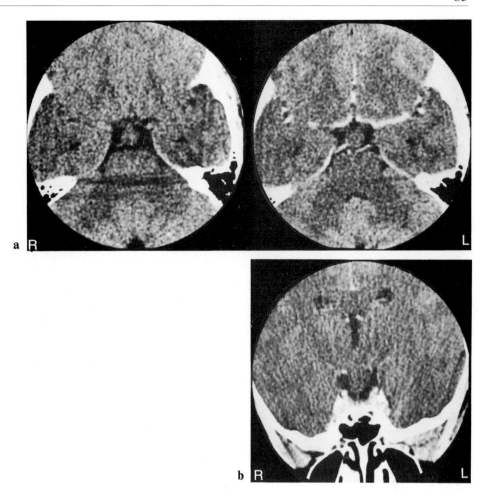

Fig. 6.22. Hypothalamic Hamartoma. An 11-year-old female. The child first had a convulsive seizure at the age of 3 years; 4 years later she had a painful swelling in the left breast and a physician was consulted. A brain CT scan revealed what was suspected to be a tumor and the patient was referred to our clinic. Upon admission, she was polyuric, but the neurological examination revealed neither visual disturbances nor a visual field defect.

a, b *CT scan.* An isodensity mass is seen in the posterior portion of the suprasellar cistern. The injection of a contrast medium produced no enhancement of the mass.

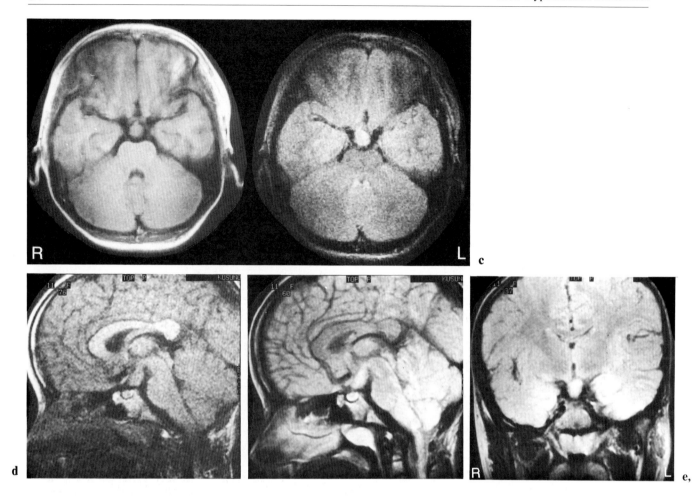

c–f *MRI*. The mass is shown as an isointensity signal in the T$_1$ weighted image and as a high intensity on the T$_2$ weighting. In the sagittal plane, it appears to emerge from between the tuber cinereum and mamillary bodies. Based on the CT and MRI findings, the diagnosis was a hypothalamic hamartoma.

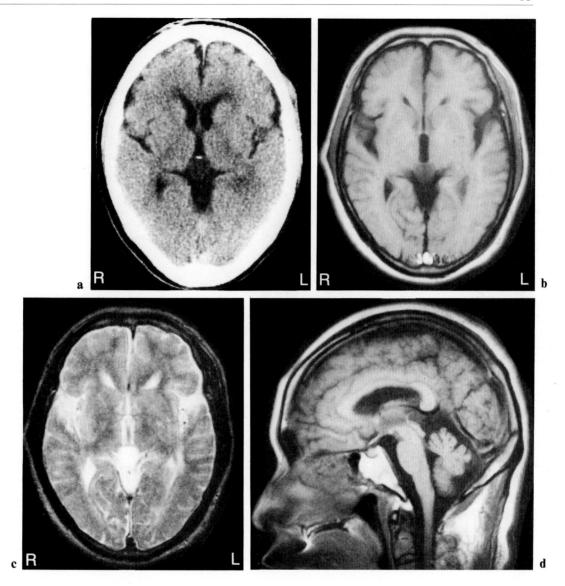

Fig. 6.23. Pineal Cyst. A 58-year-old male. The patient sought medical consultation at a hospital because of a speech disturbance and impaired hearing acuity. The case history revealed that he had been having convulsive seizures since childhood. Parinaud's sign was negative. The light reflexes were prompt and complete.

a *CT scan.* A low density area is seen in the pineal region.

b–d *MRI.* There is a low signal intensity area in the pineal region in the T_1 weighted image, but the same area is shown as a round, high signal intensity mass with a distinct margin in the T_2 weighted image. In addition, lacunae are seen within the left basal ganglia. The mass is suspected to be a pineal cyst on the basis of both the CT and MRI findings.

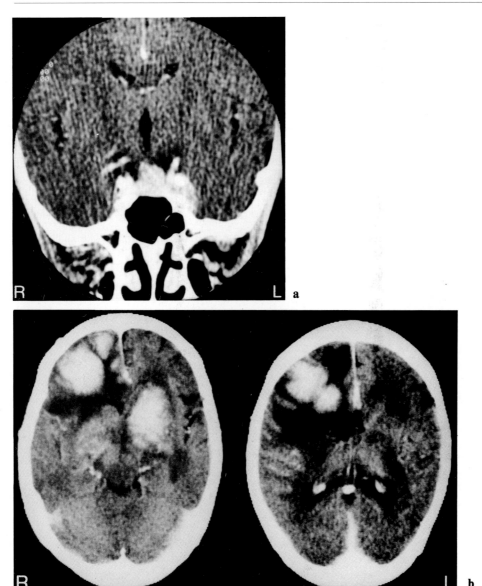

Fig. 6.24. Malignant Lymphoma. A 72-year-old female. The patient was admitted to our hospital with complaints of headache and drooping of the left eyelid. Physical examination revealed left ptosis, anisocoria (left greater than right), disturbance of lateral gaze of the left eye, sensory disturbance involving the first division of the trigeminal nerve, and a positive Barré's sign. Her level of consciousness gradually deteriorated during hospitalization.

a, b *CT scan.* Several masses are seen extending from the intrasellar region into the cavernous sinus, right frontal region, and basal ganglia, and the images are enhanced following a contrast injection. There is marked peritumoral edema.

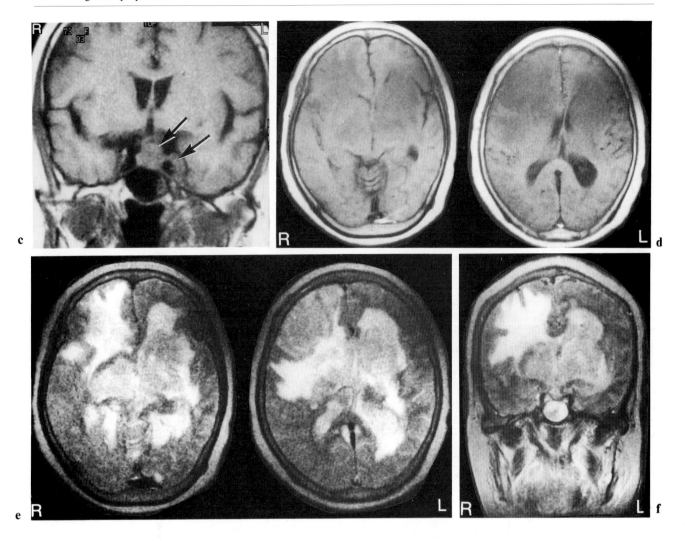

c–f *MRI.* The lesions are seen as isointense areas in the T_1 weighted image (arrows) and as iso to high intensity in the T_2 weighted image. Peritumoral edema is well demonstrated in the T_2 weighted image. The pathological study of a biopsy specimen of tumor taken from the frontal lobe was diagnosed as malignant lymphoma.

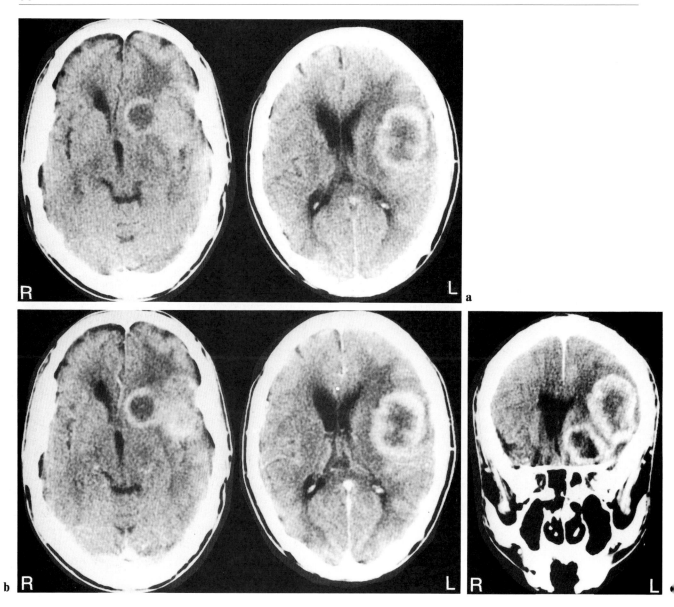

Fig. 6.25. Metastatic Brain Tumor. A 70-year-old male. Six years previously the patient had undergone surgery for thyroid cancer (histologically confirmed as papillary adenocarcinoma). Two months before consultation he developed headaches and dysarthria, and started to vomit about 1 month later. Shortly afterwards he developed a right hemiparetic gait. Upon admission, a neurological examination confirmed right hemiplegia and aphasia.

a–c *CT scan.* Multiple lesions are seen in the temporal and frontal lobes. The injection of a contrast medium produced an enhanced image. There is remarkable mass effect with perifocal edema.

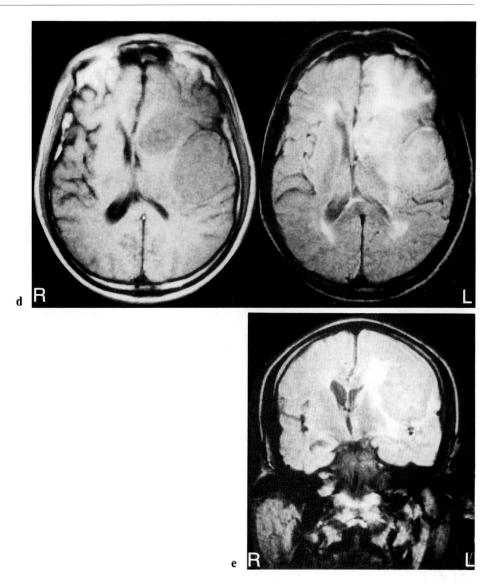

d, e *MRI.* The tumor is seen as a low signal intensity area in the T_1 weighted image and an iso to high signal intensity in T_2. Perifocal edema is shown as a high signal intensity in T_2. The MRI findings of metastatic brain tumors are similar to those of gliomas. Although perifocal edema is well-demonstrated on T_2 weighting, an enhanced CT is superior in demonstrating this type of tumor. However, MRI is superior in the demonstration of intratumoral hemorrhages, necroses, and cysts.

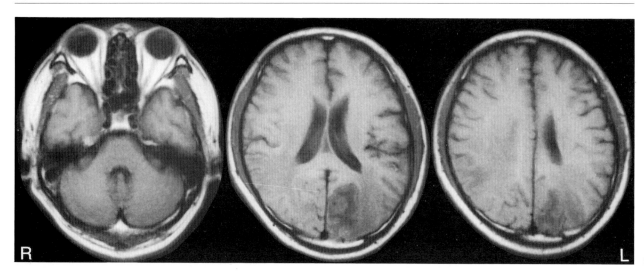

Fig. 6.26. Metastatic Brain Tumor. A 45-year-old male. Five years earlier, the patient had undergone an operation for lung cancer which had been discovered during a routine medical check-up. The surgery consisted of a left upper lobectomy and the excised tissue was histologically diagnosed as adenocarcinoma. Three years ago, a metastatic brain tumor in the left frontoparietal region was diagnosed and excised, and the patient received radiotherapy and chemotherapy. He recently developed cerebellar ataxia.

a–c *MRI.* Some enhanced masses are seen in the cerebellar hemisphere, and in the insula, left occipital, and parietal regions. Diffuse edema is seen as high intensity in the T_2 weighted image.

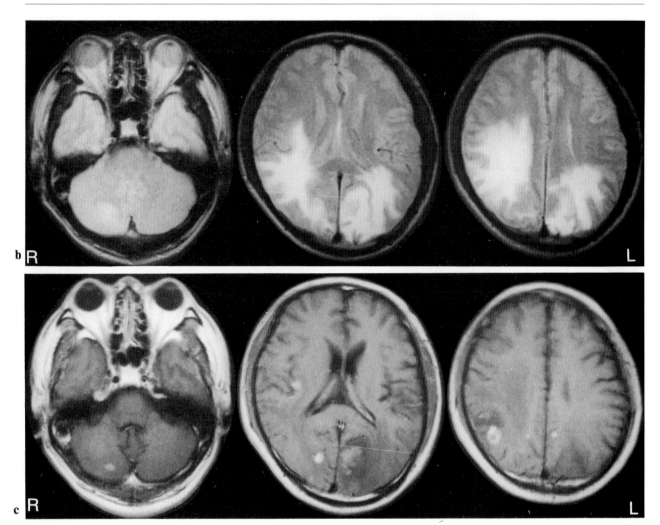

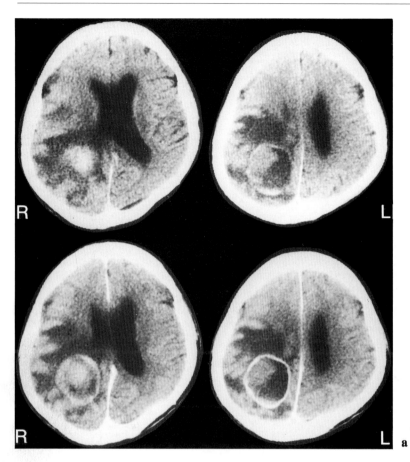

Fig. 6.27. Metastatic Brain Tumor. A 54-year-old male. Three years ago, the patient had undergone a left nephrectomy for renal carcinoma. One week prior to consultation, he developed a visual field defect and a left hemiparesis. A brain CT scan was performed and showed an abnormality. Upon admission, a neurological examination revealed a left homonymous hemianopsia and a left hemiparesis. There was no papilledema.

a *CT scan.* A ring-enhanced mass is seen in the parieto-occipital region in which a high density area suggests intratumoral hemorrhage. There is marked perifocal edema and mass effect.

b–d *MRI.* A high intensity mass is present in the left parieto-occipital region in both T_1 and T_2 weighted images. The mass shows a fluid level whose upper layer gives a high signal. The lower part has a low signal intensity. The former may represent methemoglobin which has emerged from the red cells, and the latter, deoxyhemoglobin within the red cells which have gravitated downwards. Perifocal edema is shown as a high signal intensity in the T_2 weighted image. The diagnosis of intratumoral hemorrhage was made based on the CT and MRI findings.

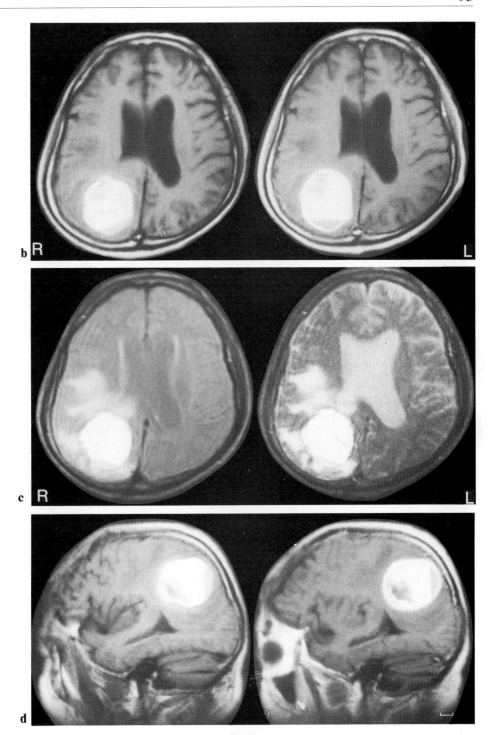

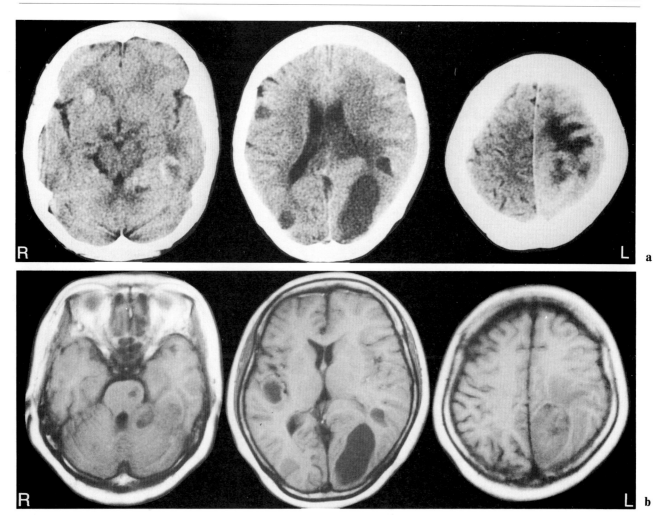

Fig. 6.28. Metastatic Brain Tumor. A 53-year-old female. The patient had undergone surgery for breast cancer 7 years ago. A few months ago, she developed a visual field defect and right hemihypesthesia with hemiparesis. The symptoms progressed rapidly and she consulted a doctor who discovered a tumor on brain CT scan and referred her to our clinic.

a, c, e *CT scan.* In the plain axial CT scan, a homogeneously high density mass is seen in the right caudate nucleus. A high density mass with a central low density area is also seen in the left temporal lobe and cerebellar hemisphere, and there are small low density masses in the temporal, frontal and occipital lobes. A slightly high density mass partly containing low density and surrounded by perifocal edema is also seen in the left parietal lobe. On contrast infusion, there is enhancement of a slightly high density portion of the mass containing a low density within it. In the contrast CT coronal section, low density areas suggesting central necrosis are seen in the right temporal, left parasagittal parietal, and occipital lobes.

b, d, f–h *MRI.* Although slice levels are somewhat different from those of CT, in T_1 weighted axial images metastatic foci of low intensity appear, one in the pons, one in the cerebellum, one each in the right temporal and occipital lobes, and one each in the occipital, temporal, and parietal lobes. In the T_2 weighted image, these foci are demonstrated more clearly with good contrast. Three foci can be identified in the cerebellum. Perifocal edema of the mass in the left parietal region is well demonstrated.

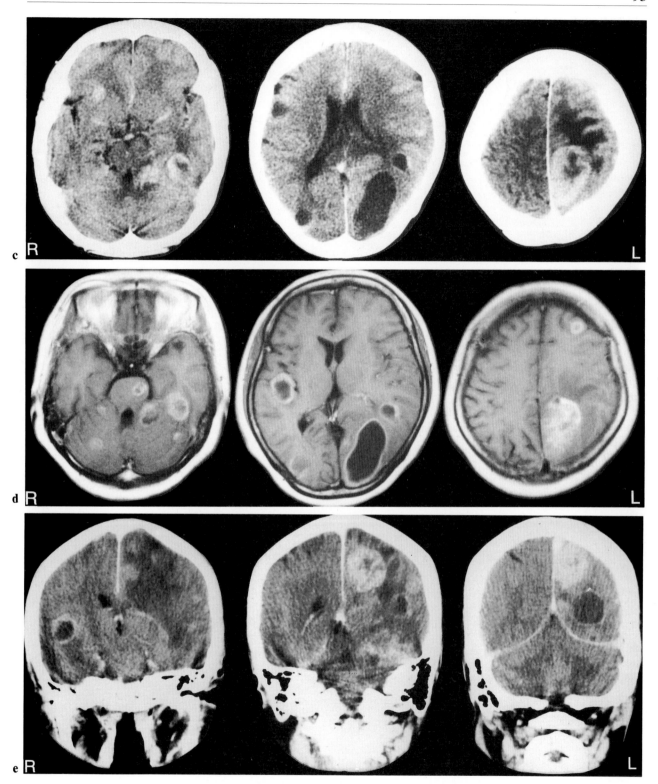

In the T_1 weighted image enhanced with Gd-DTPA, the foci are increased in number: four in the cerebellar hemisphere, two in the pons, and one small mass in the left frontal lobe. Since there was no indication for surgery, the patient was placed on chemotherapy, and referred to the radiology department for radiotherapy.

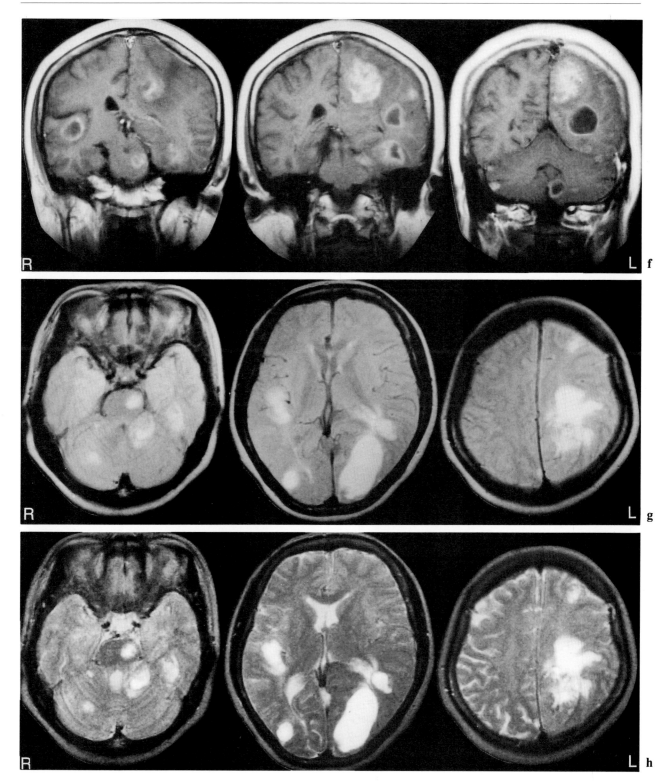

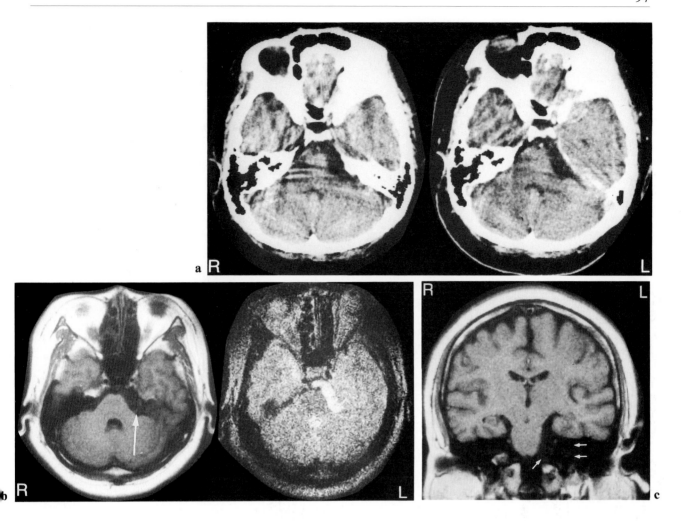

Fig. 6.29. Cerebellopontine Angle Epidermoid. A 40-year-old female. The patient had first experienced left facial pain about 14 years ago, and had only recently sought medical attention because the pain had become unbearable. The neurological examination was unremarkable except for some facial tenderness in the region of the second and third divisions of the trigeminal nerve.

a *CT scan.* A low density area is seen in the cerebellopontine angle cistern which is not clarified by the injection of contrast medium.

b, c *MRI.* A well-circumscribed low signal intensity area corresponding to that seen on CT appears in the region of the left cerebellopontine angle in the T_1 weighted image and as a high signal intensity in the T_2 weighted image. Because the signal intensity of the lesion is lower than that of CSF on T_1 and higher than that of CSF on T_2, it is possible to differentiate it from an arachnoid cyst. The tumor was removed through a lateral suboccipital approach and histologically confirmed to be an epidermoid.

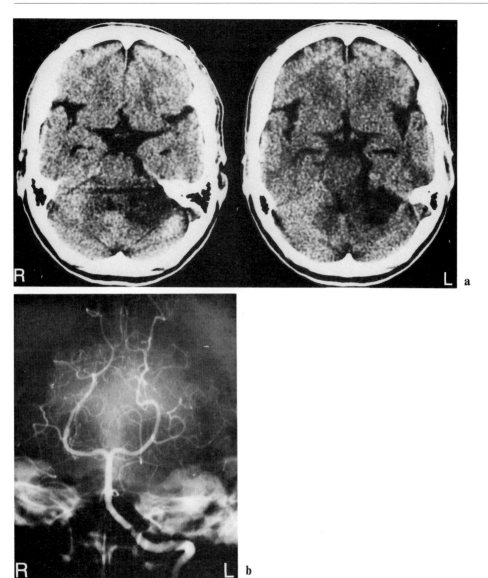

Fig. 6.30. Acoustic Neurinoma. A 57-year-old female. There was a 4-year history of hearing disturbance, and tinnitus had been present for 2–3 years. Examination upon admission was unremarkable except for decreased hearing acuity in the left ear.

a *CT scan.* A low density area is seen in the left cerebellopontine angle on the plain scan. There is a strong mass effect with displacement to the right of the fourth ventricle. Contrast material was not injected.

b *Angiography.* Specific angiographic findings include upward displacement of the left anterior cerebellar artery and the presence of a hypo- or avascular mass seen in the capillary phase.

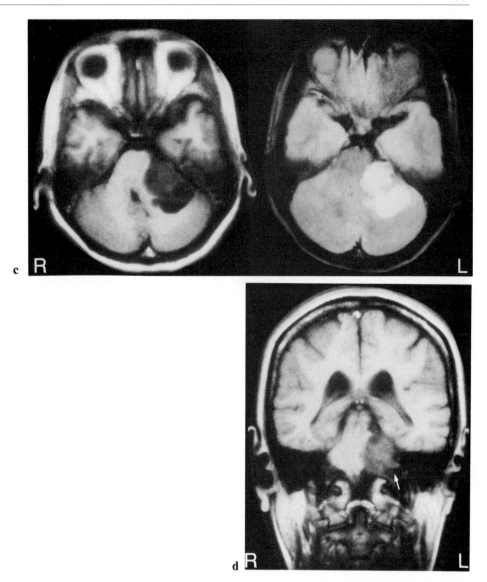

c, d *MRI*. A low signal intensity mass in the T_1 weighted image which appears as a high signal intensity on the T_2 weighting is seen in an area corresponding to that of the lesion seen on CT. The mass has a clear margin with a good demonstration of its cystic and solid components including the surrounding structures. Parts of entrapped arachnoid space are observed posterior to the tumor. The coronal image shows extension of the tumor from the auditory meatus into the cerebellopontine angle with compression of the brainstem. MRI is superior to CT in demonstrating the VIIth and VIIIth cranial nerves, the relations of tumors to these nerves, and the tentorium and fine structures within the tumor.

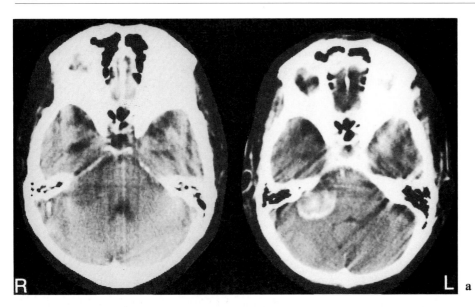

Fig. 6.31. Acoustic Neurinoma. A 65-year-old female. During admission for schizo-phrenia, the patient developed dementia. A brain CT scan revealed abnormalities and the patient was referred to our department.

a *CT scan.* A low density area is seen in the right CP angle which is homogeneously enhanced when a contrast medium is injected.

b, c *MRI.* The tumor appears as a low signal intensity in the T_1 weighted image and as a high signal intensity in the T_2 weighted image. It is well circumscribed and contains no cystic component. Ventricular enlargement with periventricular high intensity (PVHI) is present. At surgery the tumor was diagnosed as an acoustic neurinoma.

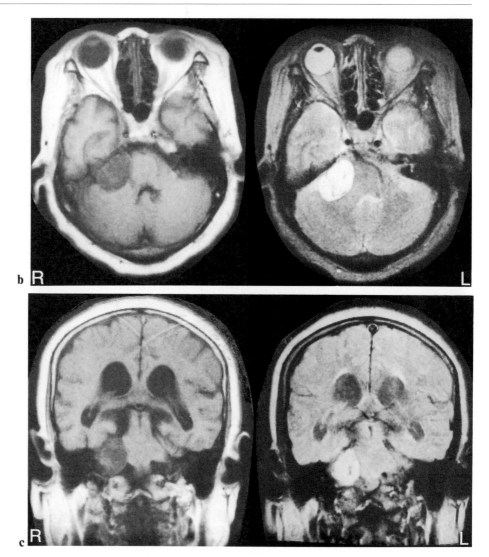

Bibliography

Albert A, Lee BCP, Saint-Louis L, Deck MDF (1986) MRI of optic chiasm and optic pathways. AJNR 7: 255–258

Araki T, Inouye T, Suzuki H, Machida T, Iio M (1984) Magnetic resonance imaging of brain tumors: measurement of T_1. Radiology 150: 95–98

Atlas SW, Grossman RI, Gomori JM, Hackney DB, Goldberg HI, Zimmerman RA, Bilaniuk LT (1987) Hemorrhagic intracranial malignant neoplasms: spin-echo MR imaging. Radiology 164: 71–77

Atlas SW, Kemp SS, Rorke L, Grossman RI (1988) Hemorrhagic intracranial retinoblastoma metastases: MR-pathology correlation. JCAT 12: 286–289

Berry I, Brant-Zawadzki M, Osaki L, Brasch R, Murovic J, Newton TH (1986) Gd-DPTA in clinical MR of the brain: 2. extraaxial lesions and normal structures. AJNR 7: 789–793

Bilaniuk LT, Zimmerman RA, Wehrli FW, Synder PJ, Goldberg HI, Grossman RI, Bottomley PA, Edelstein WA (1984) Magnetic resonance imaging of pituitary lesions using 1.0 to 1.5 T field strength. Radiology 153: 415–418

Bradac GB, Ferszi R, Bender A, Schorner W (1986) Peritumoral edema in meningiomas. A radiological and histological study. Neuroradiology 28: 304–312

Bradac GB, Schorner W, Bender A, Felix R (1985) MRI (NMR) in the diagnosis of brainstem tumors. Neuroradiology 27: 208–213

Brant-Zawadzki M, Kelly W (1986) Brain tumors. In: Brant-Zawadzki M, Norman D (eds) Magnetic resonance imaging of the central nervous system. Raven Press, New York, pp151–185

Brant-Zawadzki M, Badami JP, Mills CM, Norman D, Newton TH (1984) Primary intracranial tumor imaging: a comparison of magnetic resonance and CT. Radiology 150: 435–440

Breger RK, Papke RA, Pojunas KW, Haughton VM, Williams AL, Daniels DL (1987) Benign extraaxial tumors: contrast enhancement with Gd-DTPA. Radiology 163: 427–429

Bydder GM (1985) Magnetic resonance imaging on the posterior fossa. In Kressel HY (ed) Magnetic resonance annual 1985. Raven Press, New York, pp1–26

Bydder GM, Kingsley DPE, Brown J, Niendorf HP, Young IR (1985) Magnetic resonance imaging of meningiomas including studies with and without gadolinium-DTPA. JCAT 9: 690–697

Carr DH, Brown J, Bydder GM, Steiner RE, Weinmann HJ, Speck U, Hall AS, Young IR (1984) Intravenous chelated gadolinium as a contrast agent in NMR imaging of cerebral tumors. Lancet 1: 484–486

Claussen C, Laniado M, Kazner E, Schorner W, Felix R (1985) Application of contrast agents in CT and MRI (NMR): their potential in imaging on brain tumors. Neuroradiology 27: 164–171

Claussen C, Laniado M, Schorner W, Niendorf HP, Weinmann HJ, Fiegler W, Felix R (1985) Gadolinium-DTPA in MR imaging of glioblastomas and intracranial metastases. AJNR 6: 669–674

Colombo N, Berry I, Kucharczyk J, Kucharczyk W, de Groot J, Larson T, Norman D, Newton TH (1987) Posterior pituitary gland: appearance on MR images in normal and pathologic states. Radiology 165: 481–485

Curati WL, Graif M, Kingsley DP, King T, Scholtz CL, Steiner RE (1986) MRI in acoustic neuroma: a review of 35 patients. Neuroradiology 28: 208–214

Curati WL, Graif M, Kingsley DPE, Niendorf HP, Young IR (1986) Acoustic neurinomas: Gd-DTPA enhancement in MR imaging. Radiology 158: 447–451

Curnes JT, Lster DW, Ball MR, Moody DM, Witcofski RI (1986) MRI of radiation injury of the brain. AJR 147: 119–124

Daniels DL, Herfkens R, Koehler PR, Millen SJ, Shaffer KA, Williams AL, Haughton VM (1984) Magnetic resonance imaging of the internal auditory canal. Radiology 151: 105–108

Daniels DL, Millen SJ, Meyer GA, Pojunas KW, Kilgore DP, Shaffer KA, Williams AL, Haughton VM (1987) MR detection of tumor in the internal auditory canal. AJNR 8: 249–252

Daniels DL, Pech P, Mark L, Pojunas K, Williams AL, Haughton VM (1985) Magnetic resonance imaging of the cavernous sinus. AJR 144: 1009–1014

Daniels DL, Pech P, Pojunas KW, Kilgore DP, Williams AL, Haughton VM (1986) Trigeminal nerve: anatomic correlation with MR imaging. Radiology 159: 577–583

Daniels DL, Pojunas KW, Kilgore DP, Pech P, Meyer GA, Williams AL, Haughton VM (1986) MR of the diaphragma sellae. AJNR 7: 765–769

Daniels DL, Schenck JF, Foster T, Hart H Jr, Millen SJ, Meyer GA, Pech P, Shaffer KA, Haughton VM (1985) Surface coil magnetic resonance imaging of the internal auditory canal. AJR 145: 469–472

Davidson HD, Ouchi T, Steiner RE (1985) NMR imaging of congenital intracranial germinal layer neoplasms, Neuroradiology 27: 301–303

Dooms GC, Hecht S, Brant-Zawadzki M, Berthiaume Y, Norman D, Newton TH (1986) Brain radiation lesions: MR imaging. Radiology 158: 149–155

Dwyer AJ, Frank JA, Doppman JL, Oldfield EH, Hickey AM, Cutler GB, Loriaux DL, Schiable TF (1987) Pituitary adenomas in patients with Cushing's disease: initial experience with Gd-DTPA enhanced MR imaging. Radiology 163: 421–426

Enzmann DR, O'Donohue J (1987) Optimization MR imaging for detecting small tumors in the cerebellopontine angle and internal auditory canal. AJNR 8: 99–106

Fasano VA, Urcioli R, Ponzio RM, Lanotte MM (1986) The effects of new technologies on the surgical management of brain stem tumors. Surg Neurol 25: 219–226

Freeman MP, Kessler RM, Allen JH, Price AC (1987) Craniopharyngioma: CT and MR imaging in nine cases. JCAT 11: 810–814

Fujisawa I, Asato R, Nishimura K, Togashi K, Itoh K, Nakano Y, Itoh H, Hashimoto N, Takeuchi J, Torizuka K (1987) Anterior and posterior lobes of the pituitary gland: assessment by 1.5 T MR imaging. JCAT 11: 214–220

Fujisawa I, Kikuchi K, Nishimura K, Togashi K, Itoh K, Noma S, Minami S, Sagoh T, Hiraoka T, Momoi T, Mikawa H, Nakano Y, Itoh H, Konishi J (1987) Transection of the pituitary stalk: development of an ectopic posterior lobe assessed with MR imaging. Radiology 165: 487–489

Fujisawa I, Nishimura K, Asato R, Togashi K, Itoh K, Noma S, Kawamura Y, Sagoh T, Minami S, Nakano Y, Itoh H, Torizuka K (1987) Posterior lobe of the pituitary in diabetes insipidus: MR imaging. JCAT 11: 221–225

Fukui K, Sadamoto K, Miki H, Sakaki S, Matsuoka K (1988) Evaluation of the MRI Gd-DTPA enhancement in the diagnosis of brain and spinal tumors. Progress in Computerized Tomography 10:81–92 (English abstract)

Gentry LR, Jacoby CG, Turski PA, Houston LW, Strother CM, Sackett JF (1987) Cerebellopontine angle-petromastoid mass lesions: comparative study of diagnosis with MR imaging and CT. Radiology 162: 513–520

Glaser B, Sheinfeld M, Bonmair J, Kaplan N (1986) Magnetic resonance imaging of the pituitary gland. Clin Radiol 37: 9–14

Gomori JM, Grossman RI, Shields JA, Augsburger JJ, Joseph PM, DeSimeone D (1986) Choroidal melanomas: correlation of NMR spectrosocpy and MR imaging. Radiology 158: 443–445

Graif M, Pennock JM (1986) MR imaging of histiocytosis X in the central nervous system. AJNR 7: 21–23

Graif M, Bydder GM, Steiner RE, Niendorf P, Thomas DGT, Young IR (1985) Contrast-enhanced MR imaging of malignant brain tumors. AJNR 6: 855–862

Hahn FJ, Leibrock LG, Huseman CA, Makos MM (1988) The MR appearance of hypothalamic hamartoma. Neuroradiology 30: 65–68

Hahn FJ, Ong E, McComb RD, Mawk JR, Leibrock LG (1986) MR imaging of ruptured intracranial dermoid. JCAT 10: 888–889

Han JS, Huss RG, Benson JE, Kaufman B, Yoon YS, Morrison SC, Alfidi RJ, Rekate HL, Ratcheson RA (1984) MR imaging of the skull base. JCAT 8: 944–952

Haughton VM (1985) Magnetic resonance imaging of the cavernous sinus. AJR 144: 1009–1014

Heafner MD, Schut L, Packer RJ, Bruce DA, Bilaniuk LT, Sutton LN (1985) Discrepancy between computed tomography and magnetic resonance imaging in a case of medulloblastoma. Neurosurgery 17: 487–489

Healy ME, Hesselink JR, Press GA, Middleton MS (1987) Increased detection of intracranial metastases using intravenous gadolinium-DTPA. Radiology 165: 619–624

Hinshaw DB Jr, Fahmy JL, Peckham N, Thompson JR, Hasso AN, Holshouser B, Paprocki T (1988) The bright choroid plexus on MR: CT and pathologic correlation. AJNR 9: 483–486

Holland BA, Kucharczyk W, Brant-Zawadzki M, Norman D, Haas DK, Harper PS (1985) MR imaging of calcified intracranial lesions. Radiology 157: 353–356

House JW, Waluch V, Jackler RK (1986) Magnetic resonance imaging in acoustic neurinoma diagnosis. Ann Otol Rhinol Laryngol 95: 16–20

Hueftle MG, Han JS, Kaufman B, Berson JE (1985) MR imaging of brainstem gliomas. JCAT 9: 263–267

Just M, Higer HP, Gutjahr P, Pfannenstiel P (1986) MRI studies after treatment of brain tumors in childhood and adolescence. Child's Nerv Syst 2: 121–125

Karnaze MG, Sartor K, Winthrop JD, Gado MH, Hodges FJ III (1986) Suprasellar lesions: evaluation with MR imaging. Radiology 161: 77–82

Kean DM, Smith MA, Douglas RHB, Best JJ (1985) Two examples of CNS lipomas demonstrated by computed tomography and low field (0.08 T) MR imaging. JCAT 9: 494–496

Kelly WM, Kucharczyk W, Kucharczyk J, Kjos B, Peck WW, Norman D, Newton TH (1988) Posterior pituitary ectopia: an MR feature of pituitary dwarfism. AJNR 9: 453–460

Kilgore DP, Strother CM, Starshak RJ, Haughton VM (1986) Pineal germinoma: MR imaging. Radiology 158: 435–438

Kingsley DPE, Brooks GB, Leung AWL, Johnson MA (1985) Acoustic neuromas: evaluation by magnetic resonance imaging. AJNR 6: 1–5

Kjos BO, Brant-Zawadzki M, Kucharczyk W, Kelly WM, Norman D, Newton TH (1985) Cystic intracranial lesions of magnetic resonance imaging. Radiology 155: 363–369

Koehler PR, Haughton VM, Daniels DL, Williams AL, Yetkin Z, Charles HC, Shutts D (1985) MR measurement of normal and pathologic brainstem diameters. AJNR 6: 625–630

Koening H, Lenz M, Sauter R (1986) Temporal bone region: high resolution MR imaging using surface coils. Radiology 159: 191–194

Kucharczyk W, Brant-Zawadzki M, Sobel D, Edwards MB, Kelly WM, Norman D, Newton TH (1985) Central nervous system tumors in children: detection by magnetic resonance imaging. Radiology 155: 131–136

Kucharczyk W, Davis DO, Kelly WM, Sze G, Norman D, Newton TH (1986) Pituitary adenomas: high-resolution MR imaging at 1.5 T. Radiology 161: 761–765

Lansford LD, Martinez AJ, Latchaw RE (1987) Magnetic resonance imaging does not define tumor boundaries. Acta Radiol (Suppl) 3669: 154–156

Laster DW, Ball MR, Moody DM, Witcofski RL, Kelly DL Jr (1984) Results of nuclear magnetic resonance with cerebral glioma. Comparison with computed tomography. Surg Neurol 22: 113–122

Latack JT, Kartush JM, Kemink JL, Graham MD, Knake JE (1985) Epidermoidomas of the cerebellopontine angle and temporal bone: CT and MR aspects. Radiology 157: 361–866

Le Bas JF, Leviel JL, Decorpus M (1984) NMR relaxation times from serial stereotactic biopsies in human brain tumors. JCAT 8: 1048–1057

Lee BCP, Deck MDF (1985) Sellar and juxtasellar lesion. Detection with MR. Radiology 157: 143–147

Lee BCP, Kneeland JB, Cahill PT, Deck MDF (1985) MR recognition of supratentorial tumors. AJNR 66: 871–878

Lee BCP, Kneeland JB, Deck MDF, Cahill PT (1984) Posterior fossa lesions: magnetic resonance imaging. Radiology 153: 137–143

Lee BCP, Kneeland JB, Walker RW, Posner JB, Cahill PT, Deck MDF (1985) MR imaging of brain stem tumors. AJNR 6: 159–163

Lee DH, Norman D, Newton TH (1987) MR imaging of pineal cysts. JCAT 11: 586–590

Leksell L, Leksell D, Schwebel J (1985) Stereotaxis and nuclear magnetic resonance. J Neurol Psychiat 40: 14–18

Lloyd GAS, Phelps PD (1986) The demonstration of tumors of the parapharyngeal space by magnetic resonance imaging. Br J Radiol 59: 675–693

Lunsford LD, Martinez AJ, Latchaw RE (1986) Stereotaxic surgery with a magnetic resonance and computerized tomography-compatible system. J Neurosurg 64: 872–878

MacDonald HL, Bell BA, Smith MA, Kean DM, Tocher JL, Douglas RH, Miller JD, Best JJ (1986) Correlation of human NMR T_1 values measured in vivo and brain water content. Br J Radiol 59: 355–357

Machida T (1987) MRI diagnosis of brain tumor. Neurological Surgery 15: 485–492 (English abstract)

MacKay IM, Bydder GM, Young IR (1985) MR imaging of central nervous system tumors that do not display increases in T_1 or T_2. JCAT 9: 1055–1061

Mamourian AC, Towfighi J (1986) Pineal cysts: MR imaging. AJNR 7: 1081–1986

Mark L, Pech P, Daniels D, Charles C, Williams A, Haughton V (1984) The pituitary fossa: a correlative anatomic and MR study. Radiology 153: 453–457

Maslan MJ, Latach JT, Kemink JL, Graham MD (1986) Magnetic resonance imaging of temporal bone and cerebellopontine angle lesions. Arch Otolaryngol Head Neck Surg 112: 410–415

MaWhinney RR, Buckley JH, Holland IM, Worthington BS (1986) The value of magnetic resonance imaging in the diagnosis of intracranial meningiomas. Clin Radiol 37: 429–439

Mikhael MA, Ciric IS, Wolff AP (1985) Differentiation of cerebellopontine angle neurinomas and meningiomas with MR imaging. JCAT 9: 852–856

Mori K, Kamimura Y, Uchida Y, Kurisaka M, Eguchi S (1986) Large intramedullary lipoma of the cervical cord and posterior fossa. J Neurosurg 64: 974–976

Nakamura K, Asakura T, Yamamoto K, Nishizawa T, Todoroki K, Yamamoto Y, Fujimoto T, Okada A, Igata A (1984) Application of NMR-CT in the diagnosis of brain tumors: the correlation of T_1 relaxation times, Hounsfield units and histopathology. Progress in Computerized Tomography 6: 273–280 (English abstract)

Nemoto Y, Inoue Y, Fukuda T, Shakudo M, Katsuyama J, Hakuba A, Nishimura S, Onoyama Y (1988) MR appearance of Rathke's cleft cysts. Neuroradiology 30: 155–159

New PF, Bachow TB, Wismer GL, Rosen BR, Brady TJ (1985) MR imaging of the acoustic nerves and small acoustic neuromas at 0.6 T: prospective study. AJR 144: 1021–1026

Nishimura K, Fujisawa I, Togashi K, Itoh K, Nakano Y, Itoh H, Torizuka K (1986) Posterior lobe of the pituitary: identification by lack of chemical shift artifact in MR imaging. JCAT 10: 899–902

Numaguchi Y, Connolly ES, Kumra AK, Vargas EF, Gum GK, Mizushima A (1987) Computed tomography and MR imaging of thalamic neuroepithelial cysts. JCAT 11: 583–585

Oeckler R, Fink U, Mayr B (1986) Neurosurgical experience with magnetic resonance imaging in sellar lesions. Acta Neurochir (Wein) 8: 3–10

Olsen WL, Dillon WP, Kelly WM, Norman D, Brant-Zawadzki M, Newton TH (1986) MR imaging of paragangliomas. AJNR 7: 1039–1042

Oot R, New PFJ, Buonanno FS, Pykett IL, Kistle P, Delapaz R, Davis KR, Taveras JM, Brady TJ (1984) MR imaging of pituitary adenomas using a prototype resistive magnet: preliminary assessment AJNR 5: 131–137

Oot RF, New PFJ, Pile-Spellman J, Rosen BR, Shoukimas GM, Davis KR (1986) The detection of intracranial calcification by MR. AJNR 7: 801–809

Ormson MJ, Kispert DB, Sharbrough FW, Housner OW, Earnest F IV, Scheithauer BW, Laws ER Jr (1986) Cryptic structural lesions in refractory partial epilepsy: MR imaging and CT studies. Radiology 160: 215–219

Packer RJ, Batnitzky S, Cohen ME (1985) Magnetic resonance imaging in the evaluation of intracranial tumors of childhood. Cancer 57 (Suppl): 1767–1772

Packer RJ, Zimmerman RA, Bilaniuk LT (1986) Magnetic resonance imaging in the detection of neurological damage caused by treatment of childhood cancer. Ann Neurol 18: 403–485

Packer RJ, Zimmerman RA, Luerssen TG, Bruce DA, Schut L (1985) Brain stem gliomas of childhood: magnetic resonance imaging. Neurology 35: 397–401

Peterman SB, Steiner RE, Bydder GM, Thomas DJ, Tobias JS, Young IR (1985) Nuclear magnetic resonance imaging (NMR), (MRI), of brain stem tumors. Neuroradiology 27: 202–207

Potts DG, Zimmerman RD (1985) Nuclear magnetic resonance imaging of skull base lesions. Can J Neurol Sci 12: 327–331

Press GA, Hesselink JR (1988) MR imaging of cerebellopontine angle and internal auditory canal lesions at 1.5 T. AJNR 9: 241–251

Richards MA, Webb JAW, Reznek RH, Davies G, Jewell SE, Shand WS, Wrigley PFM, Lister TA (1986) Detection of spread of malignant lymphoma to the liver by low field strength magnetic resonance imaging. Br Med J 293: 1126–1128

Rinck PA, Meindl S, Higer HP, Bieler EU, Pfannenstiel P (1985) Brain tumors: detection and typing by use of CPMG sequences and in vivo T_2 measurements. Radiology 157: 103–106

Robinson DA, Steiner RE, Young IR (1988) The MR contribution after CT demonstration of supratentorial mass effect without additional localizing features. JCAT 12: 275–279

Roosen N, Gahlen D, Strok W, Neuen E, Wecksler W, Schirmer M, Lins E, Bock WJ (1987) Magnetic resonance imaging of colloid cysts of the third ventricle. Neuroradiology 29: 10–14

Sartor K, Karnaze MG, Winthrop JD, Gado M, Hodges FJ III (1987) MR imaging in infra-, para- and retrosellar mass lesions. Neuroradiology 29: 19–29

Sasaki Y, Machida T (1988) Brain tumor: supratentorial lesion. Journal of Medical Imagings 8:375–383 (Japanese)

Schoner W, Laniado M, Niendorf HP, Schubert C, Felix R (1986) Time-dependent changes in image contrast in brain tumors after gadolinium-DTPA, AJNR 7: 1013–1020

Schroth G, Gawehn J, Marquardt B, Schabet M (1986) MR imaging of esthesioneuroblastoma. JCAT 10: 316–319

Scotti G, Yu C-Y, Dillon WP, Norman D, Colombo N, Newtton TH, Groot JD, Wilson CB (1988) MR imaging of cavernous sinus involvement by pituitary adenoma. AJNR 9: 657–664

Shuman WP, Griffin BR, Haynor DR, Johnson JS, Jones DC, Cromwell LD, Moss AA (1985) MR imaging in radiation therapy planning. Radiology 156: 143–147

Smith AS, Weinstein MA, Modic MT, Pavlicek W, Rogers LR, Budd TG, Bukowski RM, Purvis JD, Weick JK, Duchesneau PM (1985) Magnetic resonance with marked T_2-weighted images improved demonstration of brain lesions, tumor and edema. AJR 145: 949–955

Snow RB, Lavyne MH, Lee BCP, Morgello S, Patterson RH (1986) Craniotomy versus transsphenoidal excision of large pituitary tumors: the usefulness of magnetic resonance imaging in guiding the operative approach. Neurosurgery 19: 59–64

Spagnoli MC, Goldberg HI, Grossman RI, Bilaniuk LT, Gomori JM, Hackney DB, Zimmerman RA (1986) Intracranial meningiomas: high-field MR imaging. Radiology 161: 369–375

Spagnoli MV, Grossman RI, Packer RJ, Hackney DB, Goldberg HI, Zimmerman RA, Bilaniuk LT (1987) Magnetic resonance imaging determination of gliomatosis cerebri. Neuroradiology 29: 15–18

Sunada S, Yamaura A, Suzuki N, Uozumi A, Okada J, Uno K, Miyoshi T, Arimizu N, Uematsu S, Morita F (1986) The effect of Gd-DTPA as a contrast agent in MR imaging: the evaluation of brain tumors. Progress in Computerized Tomography 8:267–376 (English abstract)

Suto Y, Kimura K, Okumura R, Ishii Y (1988) Pituitary adenoma and parasellar tumors. Journal of Medical Imagings 8:384–389 (Japanese)

Takahashi M, Yamashita Y, Sakamoto Y, Kojima R (1988) Posterior fossa tumors. Journal of Medical Imagings 8:405–412 (Japanese)

Thomas DGT, Davis CH, Ingram S, Olney JS, Bydder GM, Young IR (1986) Stereotaxic biopsy of the brain under MR imaging control. AJNR 7: 161–163

Tjon-A-Tham RTO, Bloem JL, Falke THM, Bijvoet OLM, Gohel VK, Harinck BIJ, Ziedses des Plantes GB Jr (1985) Magnetic resonance imaging in Paget disease of the skull. AJNR 6: 879–881

Wagle VG, Villemure JG, Melanson D, Ethier R, Bertrand G, Feindel W (1987) Diagnostic potential of magnetic resonance in cases of foramen magnum meningiomas. Neurosurgery 21: 622–626

Yagura H, Komiyama M, Fu Y, Baba M, Yasui T, Hakuba A, Nishimura S, Shakudo M, Inoue Y (1986) Diagnosis of meningioma in magnetic resonance imaging. Progress in Computerized Tomography 8:675–682 (English abstract)

Yamada K, Matsuzawa T, Yamada S, Hishinuma T, Yamada S, Yoshioka S, Ono S (1986) Magnetic resonance imaging and relaxation time studies of brain oedema. Adv Neurol Sci 30: 451–460

Yamanaka M, Uozumi T, Sakoda K, Ohta M, Kawashima K, Mukada K, Kanazawa J, Kagawa Y, Kajima T (1987) Magnetic resonance imaging of pituitary microadenomas. Progress in Computerized Tomography 9:505–512 (English abstract)

Yeakley JW, Kulkarni M, McArdle CB, Haar FL, Tang RA (1987) High-resolution MR imaging of juxtasellar meningiomas with CT and angiographic correlation. AJNR 9: 279–285

Yoshida K, Inao S, Saso K, Motegi Y, Kaneok Y, Furuse M (1987) Evaluation of peritumoral edema by proton T_1 values with special remarks to time course following intracranial surgery. Neurological Surgery 15:389–395 (English abstract)

Yuh WTC, Barloon TJ, Jacoby CG (1987) Case report. Trigeminal nerve lipoma: MR findings. JCAT 11: 518–521

Yuh WTC, Wright DC, Barloon TJ, Jacoby CG (1987) MR imaging of primary tumors of trigeminal nerve and Meckel's cave. AJNR 9: 665–670

Zimmerman RA (1985a) Magnetic resonance imaging of cerebral neoplasms. In: Kressel HY (ed) Magnetic resonance annual. Raven Press, New York, pp113–148

Zimmerman RA (1985b) Magnetic resonance imaging of midline pediatric cerebral neoplasms. Acta Neurochir Suppl 35: 60–64

Zimmerman RA, Bilaniuk LT, Packer R, Sutton L, Samuel L, Johnson MH, Grossman RI, Goldberg HI (1985) Resistive NMR of brain stem gliomas. Neuroradiology 27: 21–25

Zimmerman RD, Flemming CA, Saint-Louis LA, Lee BCP, Manning JJ, Deck MDF (1985) Magnetic resonance imaging of meningiomas. AJNR 6: 149–157

7 Cerebrovascular Disorders

Changes in red blood cell hemoglobin are reflected as changes in signal intensity on MRI, thereby allowing chronological changes in intracerebral hematomas to be easily detected. Immediately after a hemorrhage, there is an accumulation of oxyhemoglobin which is converted into deoxyhemoglobin. Oxyhemoglobin does not influence the relaxation time of hydrogen ions, but deoxyhemoglobin shortens it. Consequently, within the first few hours of a hemorrhage, a hematoma is shown with the same signal intensity as gray matter in both T_1 and T_2 weighted images. The low signal area at the periphery of the hematoma seen in a T_1 weighted image (shown as a high signal intensity on T_2) is thought to represent serum. Two to three days after the hemorrhage, a partially high intensity area may be seen on T_1 due to the presence of deoxyhemoglobin, but in the T_2 weighted image, the whole area is seen as a low signal intensity. From about the first week after the hemorrhage, hemolysis commences from the periphery, with oxidation of deoxyhemoglobin and its conversion into methemoglobin. Both in the T_1 and T_2 weighted images, the hematoma passes through the stage of iso intensity until the periphery becomes a high signal intensity area on T_1 and gradually spreads centrally. The accompanying liquefaction of the hematoma which proceeds from the periphery towards the center is also gradually shown as a high signal intensity on T_2. Formation of a hematoma capsule starts from 2–3 weeks after the hemorrhage. Methemoglobin is phagocytosed by macrophages and converted into hemosiderin, which also shortens the relaxation time. In a T_1 weighted image, the uniformly high signal intensity area changes into a low signal intensity; on T_2, liquefaction of hematoma is seen as a homogeneously high signal intensity area, and linear low signal areas appear at the periphery of the hematoma. Several months after a hemorrhage, the hematoma undergoes scar formation which is also seen as a low intensity area.

Since MRI produces no signal where there is blood flow (flow void), cerebral arteriovenous malformations (AVM), venous angiomas and other similar lesions can be diagnosed easily. Additionally, the absence of bony artifacts in the posterior cranial fossa on MRI makes it possible to detect very small lesions in the brainstem. Cerebral infarctions can be detected much earlier than on CT, being visible within hours of occurrence. Most other lesions follow the same pattern — a low signal on T_1 and a high signal on T_2 weighting. Since MRI can indicate blood flow, it can also reveal vascular obstructions resulting from thromboses. A comparatively recent blood thrombus is seen as a high signal intensity area, while an older one has a low signal intensity. The unobstructed segment appears between a signal void and a low signal intensity area. It is believed that MRI angiography will soon become a standard clinical technique.

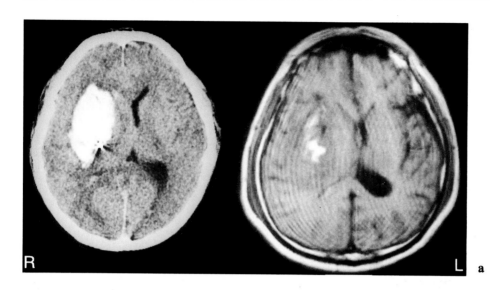

Fig. 7.1. Intracerebral Hemorrhage. A 49-year-old male. The initial symptoms included acute abdominal pain and vomiting followed immediately by rapid deterioration in the level of consciousness. Upon medical examination, the blood pressure was found to be 170/110 mmHg, and a CT scan was performed revealing a right putaminal hemorrhage. The patient was subsequently admitted to our clinic where his level of consciousness was 30 (Japan Coma Scale). He also had a right hemiparesis which was more marked in the lower extremity. On the same day, at emergency surgery, a hematoma was evacuated through a burr hole.

a, b *CT and MRI* (two days after occurrence). An irregular lesion is seen in the right basal ganglia and is associated with a remarkable mass effect. In both the T_1 and T_2 weighted images, the central part of the lesion shows a high signal intensity representing deoxymethemoglobin. The outer portion shows an iso to a low signal intensity in the T_1 weighted image, and a low intensity close to a signal void in the T_2 weighted image, representing intracellular methemoglobin. The outermost layer shows an iso to a low intensity in the T_1 weighted image and a high signal intensity in the T_2 weighted image, representing perifocal edema.

c, d *MRI* (one month after occurrence). The T_1 weighted image shows the central portion as a low to isointensity signal and the periphery as a high signal intensity. The T_2 weighted image shows the whole area as a high intensity surrounded by a zone of moderately high intensity. The perifocal region seems to be edema whereas the signal of the central portion seems to represent cystic change. There is a slight widening of the ring portion following enhancement of the image with Gd-DTPA.

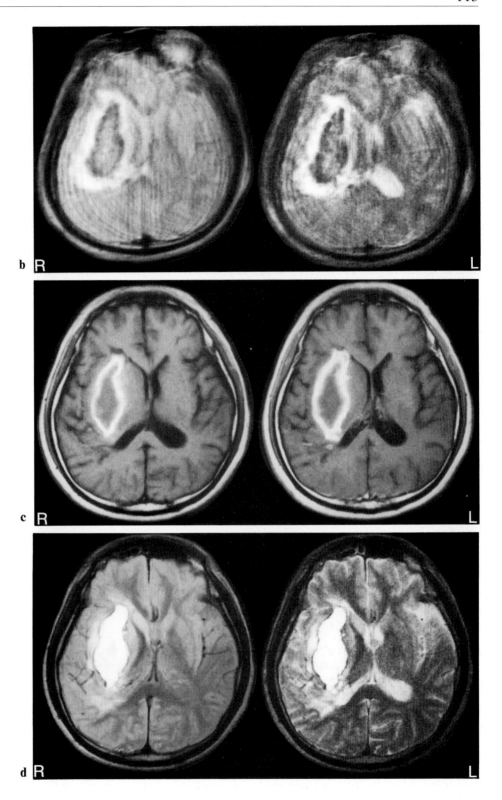

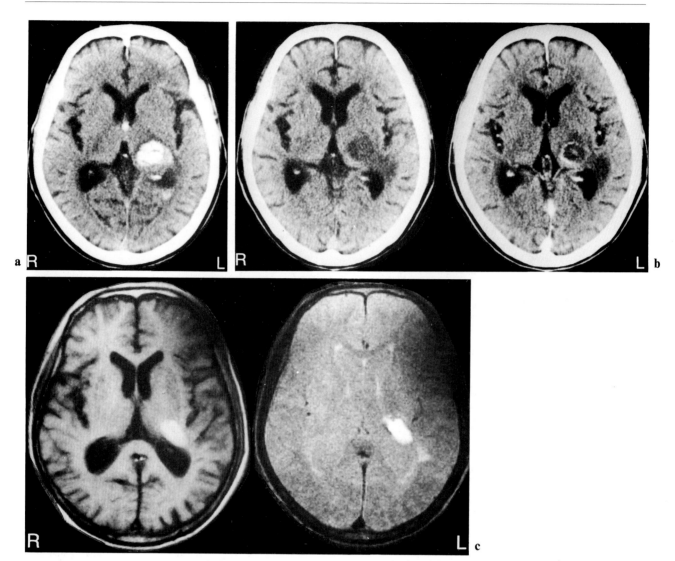

Fig. 7.2. Thalamic Hemorrhage. A 70-year-old female. The patient had suddenly developed a right hemiparesis and had fallen down while at work. She developed a dysarthria and a neurological examination at our clinic confirmed a right hemiparesis and hemihypesthesia. Blood pressure was 206/104 mmHg.

a, b *CT scan.* A brain CT scan performed upon admission revealed a hematoma in the left thalamus associated with intraventricular penetration. A month following the attack, a repeat scan showed conversion of the area of hemorrhage into a low density which was enhanced in a ring-like fashion upon injection of a contrast medium.

c *MRI.* MRI performed about 1 month following the attack showed a high signal intensity in both the T_1 and T_2 weighted images in the area corresponding to the site of the hematoma revealed on CT.

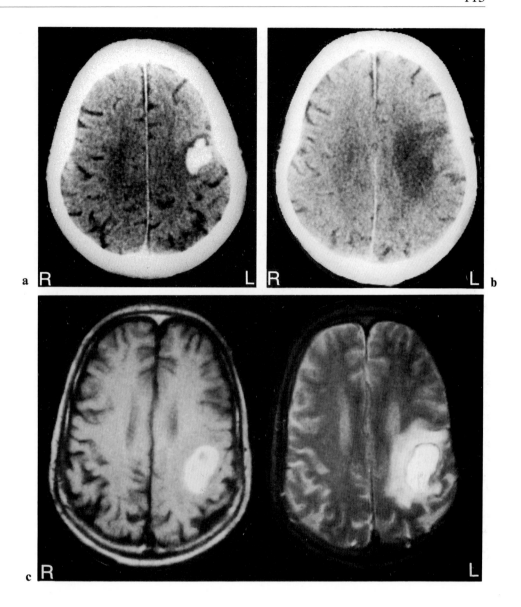

Fig. 7.3. Subcortical Hemorrhage. A 64-year-old male. The initial symptom was weakness of the right upper extremity followed by speech disturbance. Upon examination at our clinic, a slight right hemiparesis was noted. Blood pressure was 110/80 mmHg. Pertinent hematological findings included: GOT 115 IU/1, GPT 152 IU/1, ChE 180 IU/dl.

a, b *CT scan.* The admission CT scan showed a high density area measuring about 2 cm in diameter in the left parietal subcortical region. The CT examination 1 month later showed that the hematoma was absorbed and that the area had converted to a low density.

c *MRI.* On MRI performed 3 weeks later, the mass is seen as a high signal intensity in both the T_1 and T_2 weighted images. A high signal intensity around the hematoma in the T_2 image probably represents edema. The hematoma in this case may have been caused by a hemorrhagic tendency resulting in liver dysfunction.

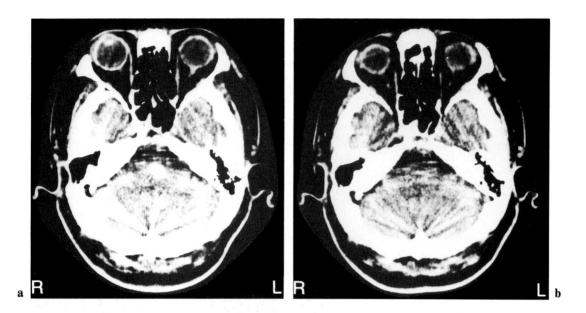

Fig. 7.4. Pontine Hemorrhage. A 69-year-old male. The patient was brought fully conscious and alert to our hospital after suddenly developing numbness in the right hand. Neurological findings included: disturbed lateral gaze of the left eye, horizontal nystagmus, right peripheral facial palsy, right hemiplegia, and a right hemisensory disturbance below the neck.

a, b *CT scan.* The CT scan upon admission showed a high density area in the midline of the pons suggestive of a pontine hemorrhage. The extent of the lesion was not clear due to the presence of bony artifact. A repeat CT 10 days after the attack failed to identify the area of the hemorrhage.

c, d *MRI.* MRI performed 8 days after the attack shows a high signal intensity in both the T_1 and T_2 weighted images. Possible edema is seen around the lesion in T_2. Unlike the CT scan, intracerebral hemorrhage cannot be demonstrated immediately after an attack on MRI. However, hemorrhage is seen as a low to isointensity signal 3 days following the attack, and as a high intensity 1 to 2 weeks in either the T_1 or T_2 weighted images as a result of the effect of methemoglobin. That is, in the T_1 weighted image, T_1 begins to shorten from the periphery of the hematoma 1 week following the episode and the lesion becomes ring-shaped. Its center also appears as high signal intensity area. Thus, MRI provides not only the diagnosis of hematoma, but also makes it possible to estimate the time interval since the occurrence (i.e., the age of the hematoma).

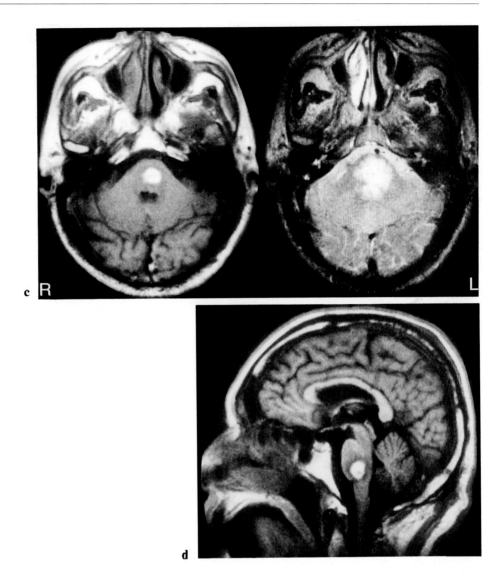

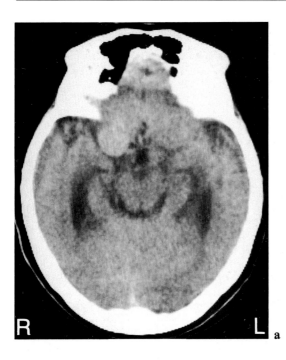

Fig. 7.5. Giant Saccular Aneurysm. A 69-year-old female. The patient lost consciousness and was brought to a nearby hospital. The CT scan revealed what was believed to be a subarachnoid hemorrhage and she was transferred to our hospital. Upon admission, the level of consciousness was estimated at 2 (Japan Coma Scale); a left hemiparesis and nuchal rigidity were present.

a *CT scan.* An isodensity area is seen in the region corresponding to the bifurcation of the right internal carotid artery. This is accompanied by ventricular dilatation.

b *Angiography.* Right carotid angiography shows a giant aneurysm at the bifurcation of the internal carotid artery.

c, d *MRI.* The mass gives no signal and was therefore suspected to be a giant aneurysm. The different signal intensities within the lesion may be due to internal turbulence.

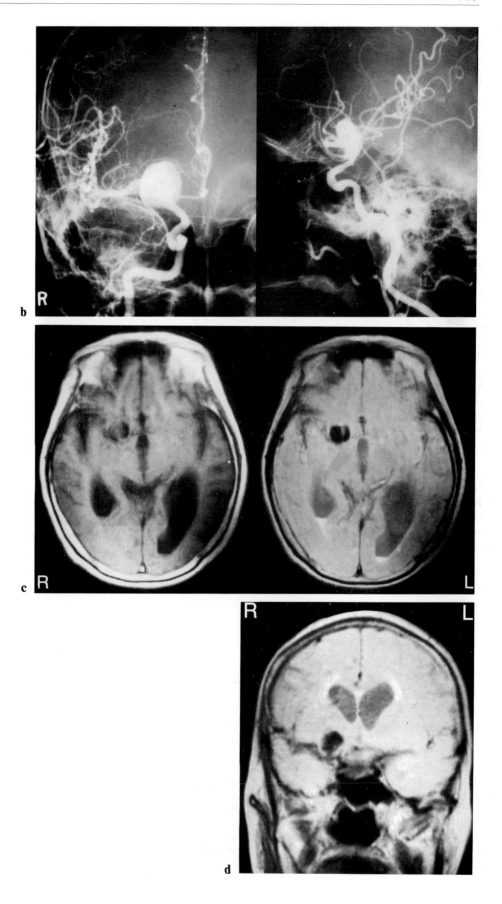

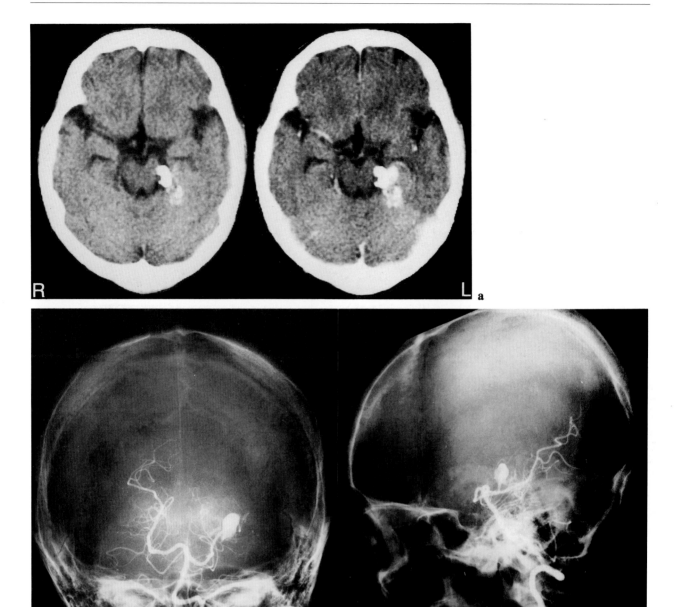

Fig. 7.6. Thrombosed Aneurysm of the Posterior Cerebral Artery. A 58-year-old female. There was a 2 month history of dizziness, heaviness of the head, and slight hemiparesis. A neurological examination confirmed left hemiparesis associated with hyperactive deep tendon reflexes.

a *CT scan.* In the plain axial CT, narrowing of the right ambient cistern and an isodensity mass with a mixture of high density possibly due to calcification is seen compressing the right cerebral peduncle and midbrain. Injection of contrast material produces some enhancement of the image.

b *Angiography.* A saccular aneurysm can be seen in the P_2–P_3 portion of the posterior cerebral artery on left vertebral angiography. The mass effect exerted on the surrounding branches suggests that the aneurysm is larger than the size indicated by the angiogram.

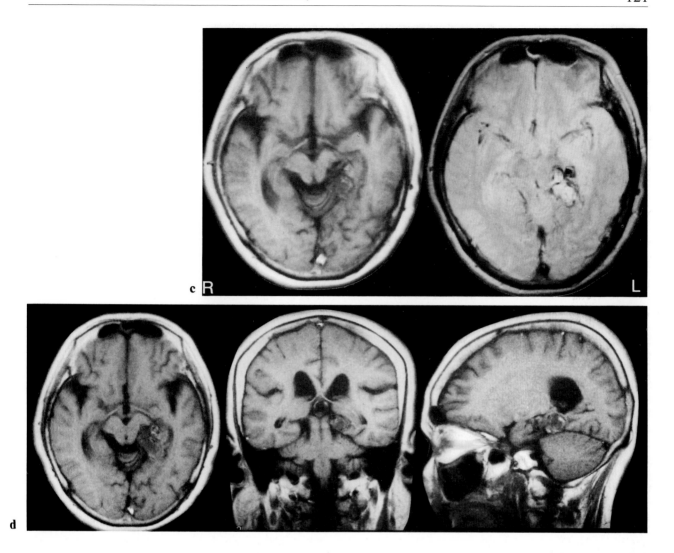

c, d *MRI.* In the T_1 weighted axial image, a mass of inhomogeneous intensity is seen in the ambient cistern compressing the right cerebral peduncle and the right side of the midbrain. The mass is for the most part shown as a slight low intensity with part of it containing a mixture of high intensity suggesting lipid and low intensity indicating calcification. The slightly low intensity part is intensified by Gd-DTPA, which is surrounded by low intensity spots of calcifications. The posterior cerebral artery and aneurysmal lumen appear as a signal void. In both the coronal and sagittal T_1 weighted images, a low intensity mass is surrounded by a slightly high intensity band representing a lipid deposit. This lesion is considered to be a thrombosed aneurysm.

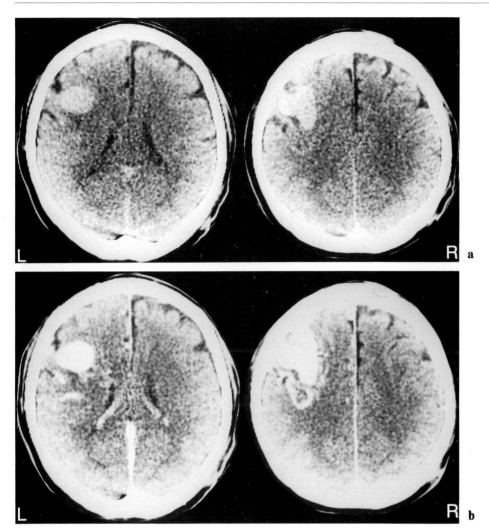

Fig. 7.7. Cerebral Arteriovenous Malformation. A 53-year-old male. Right-sided
hemiconvulsions began about 15 years prior to consultation. Minor seizures occasionally
associated with headache occurred daily in spite of anticonvulsive medications. The
physical examination was unremarkable.

a, b *CT scan.* Plain CT (**a**) reveals a homogeneous high density mass with minimal
mass effect in the left frontoparietal region, which is markedly enhanced on enhanced
CT (**b**).

c, d *Angiogram.* On left carotid angiograms (**c** anteroposterior view; **d** lateral view),
an arterio-venous malformation in the frontoparietal region is shown, which is fed by
the left central and precentral arteries and drained by the Trolard vein.

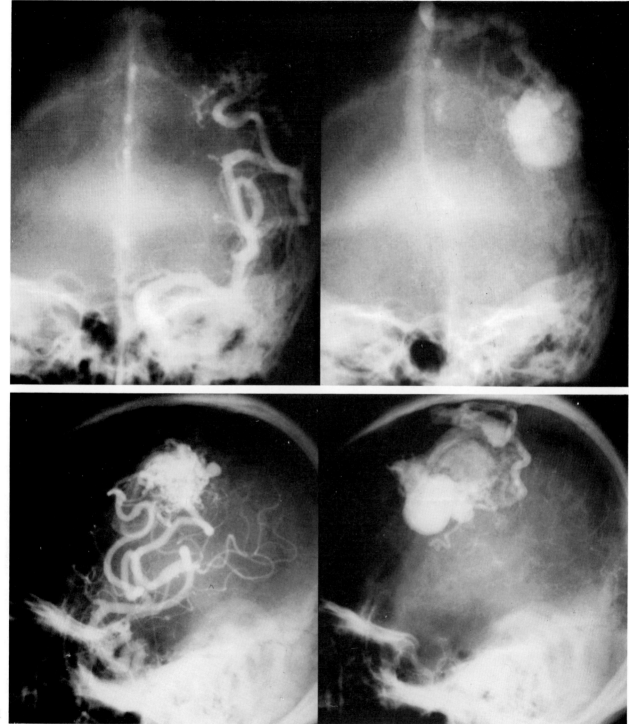

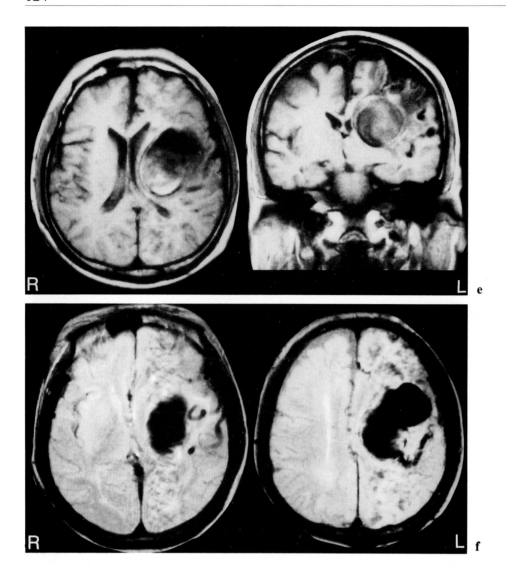

e, f *MRI.* A homogeneously high density mass with numerous vascular components can be seen in the left frontoparietal region. There are also associated phase-encoding artifacts due to a pulsating flow in the lesion. The high signal intensity seen in the lesion in the T_1 weighted image represents a mural thrombosis. The area surrounding the lesion, which is seen as a high signal intensity in the T_2 weighted image, may be the result of ischemic changes resulting from the "steal phenomenon". In high-flow AVMs, identification of the feeder, nidus, and drainer is possible without the use of contrast agents. In an AVM associated with hematoma, differentiation of the nidus from the hematoma is also possible, and the age of the hematoma can be estimated as well.

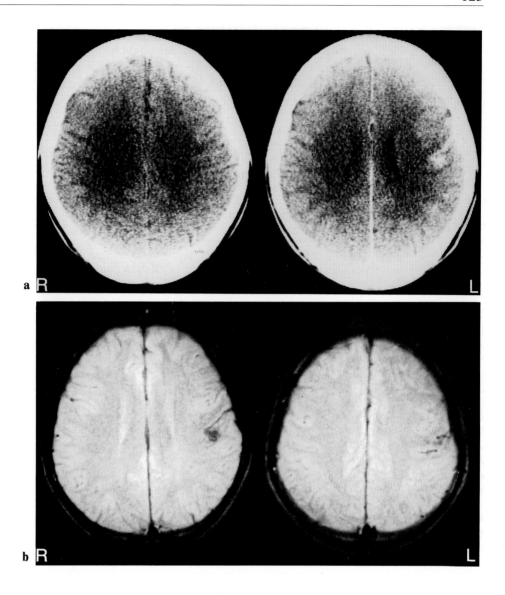

Fig. 7.8. Cerebral Arteriovenous Malformation. A 34-year-old male. The patient had developed convulsive seizures and headaches 3 days prior to consulting our service. The neurological examination was negative.

a *CT scan.* A lesion is clearly seen in the left frontoparietal region.

b *MRI.* In the same region as shown on CT, a nidus with a vascular component and a signal void is seen in the T$_2$ weighted image. There is no infarction resulting from the "steal phenomenon" around the lesion. An AVM was diagnosed from the CT and MRI findings.

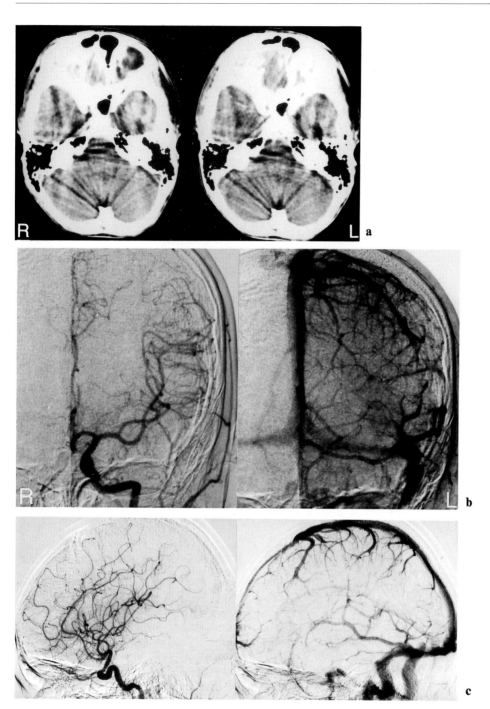

Fig. 7.9. Cavernous Angioma. A 10-year-old male. A black nevus about the size of a palm was noted at birth. Two weeks prior to consultation, the child started having headaches with attacks of nausea occurring about 2–3 times daily. The neurological examination was unremarkable.

a *CT scan.* An iso to slightly hyperdense mass is seen at the tip of the left temporal lobe, and is not enhanced by an injection of contrast medium.

b, c *Angiography.* A superomedial dislocation of the Sylvian point is seen in the anteroposterior view, and upward displacement in the lateral view. No tumor stain is present.

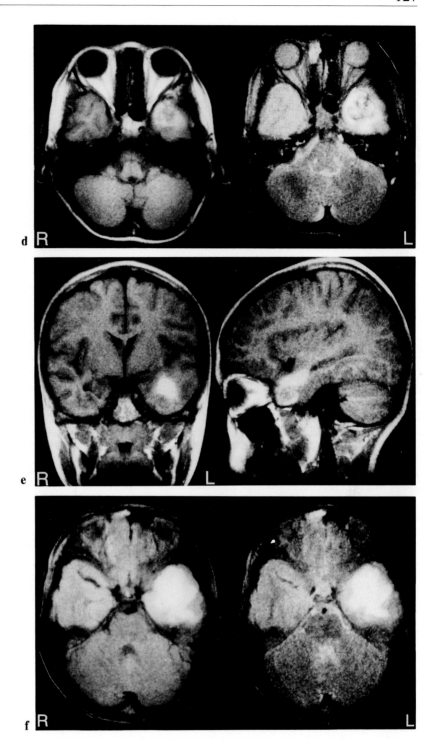

d-f *MRI*. A high signal intensity mass is seen in the left temporal tip in both the T_1 and T_2 weighted images. There is reticular formation inside the mass, and a high signal intensity area corresponding to perifocal edema is seen in the T_2 weighted image. The entire mass was removed through a left temporal craniotomy. There was a thrombus within the mass and the lesion was histologically diagnosed as a cavernous angioma.

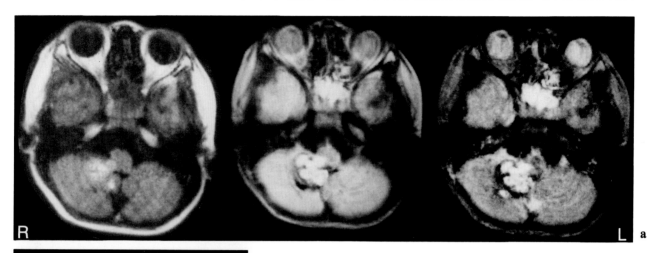

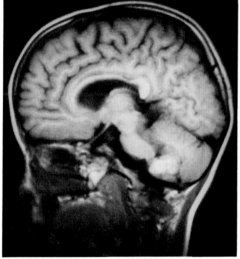

Fig. 7.10. Venous Angioma in the Cerebellum. A 4-year-old male. The child apparently fell from a height of approximately 1.5 m and struck his head on a hard surface. He was rushed to a nearby hospital where an initial CT scan revealed a cerebellar hemorrhage. He was transferred to our service where the neurological examination was unremarkable; intracranial pressure was not elevated.

a, b *MRI.* A cluster of small high signal intensity spots is seen in the right cerebellar hemisphere in both the T_1 and T_2 weighted images. This represents either a hematoma of a few months' duration or recent thrombi. In the T_2 weighted image, a flow void is seen posterior to the high intensity area, which probably represents a blood vessel. A low intensity in the dorsal part of the medulla seems to be partial volume effect due to angioma. The patient has been followed up continuously and no surgery has been performed.

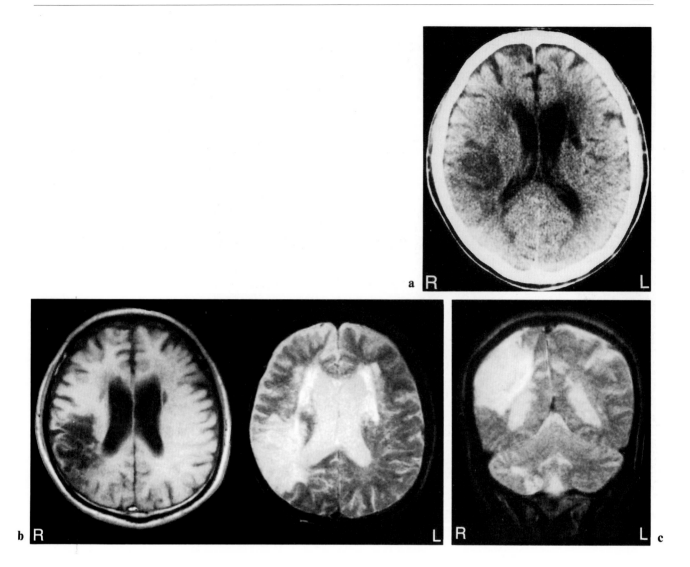

Fig. 7.11. Occlusion of the Middle Cerebral Artery. A 62-year-old male. The patient consulted us after suddenly developing weakness of the left lower extremity and speech disturbance. Upon examination, a left hemiparesis with exaggerated deep tendon reflexes as well as other pathological reflexes were present.

a *CT scan.* A low density area is seen in the territory of the right middle cerebral artery, and a lacuna is present in the paraventricular region on the left side. Carotid angiography confirmed an occlusion of the right middle cerebral artery.

b, c *MRI.* The infarct is seen as a low signal intensity area in the T₁ weighted image and as a high signal intensity in the T₂ weighted image. However, these findings are not pathognomonic of an infarct as some other pathological processes, such as demyelination and tumors, may also exhibit a similar pattern on MRI.

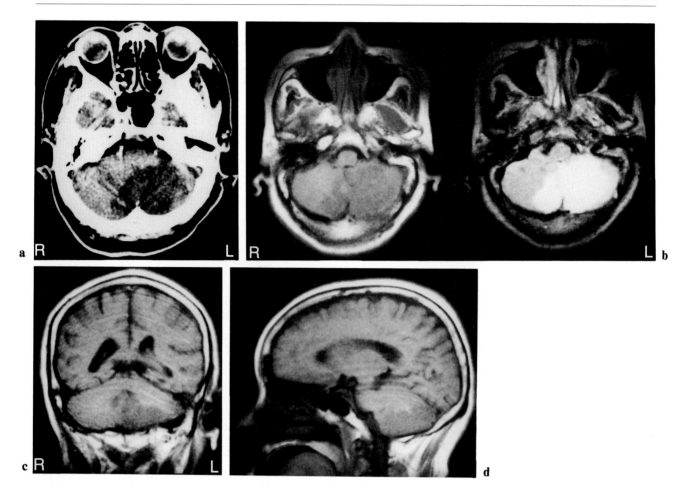

Fig. 7.12. Cerebellar Infarction. A 73-year-old female. The patient fell following a sudden attack of vertigo and was brought to the hospital. Upon admission, her blood pressure was 180/103 mmHg, the level of consciousness was 1 (Japan Coma Scale), and horizontal nystagmus and left cerebellar signs were present.

a *CT scan.* A diffuse low density area is seen in the left cerebellar hemisphere, vermis, and part of the right hemisphere.

b–d *MRI.* The area of infarct is seen as a low signal intensity in the T_1 weighted image and as a high signal intensity on T_2 weighting. In the sagittal plane, the infarct is localized in the lower half of the cerebellum. It was subsequently diagnosed as a lesion resulting from an occlusion of the anterior inferior cerebellar and posterior inferior cerebellar arteries.

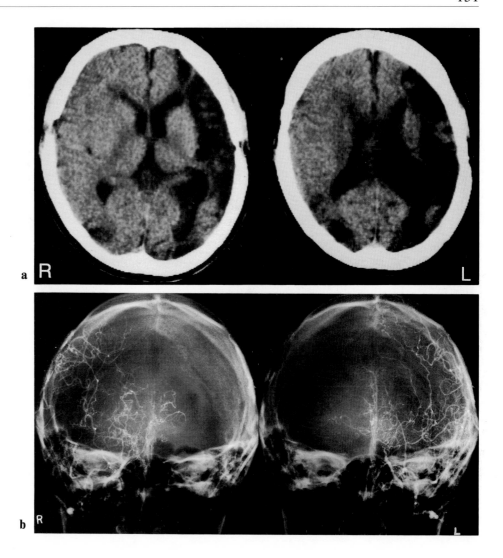

Fig. 7.13. Moyamoya Disease. A 15-year-old female. The patient developed alternating hemiplegia at 2 years of age. Encepholo-Duro-Arterio-Synangiosis (EDAS) was performed when she was 9 years old, and the medical history since then has been uneventful. There was no motor palsy upon examination; the patient is mentally retarded.

a *CT scan.* Low density areas due to infarction are seen in the left cerebral hemisphere and right occipital lobe. Asymmetry of the lateral ventricles is present.

b–d *Angiography.* Occlusion of the bifurcations of both internal carotid arteries is seen. Collateral circulation through the superficial temporal artery is present. Vault moyamoya is prominent in the left carotid angiogram, and basal moyamoya appears in the right carotid angiogram.

e–g *MRI.* Infarcts, shown as low intensity areas in the T_1 weighted image and as a high intensity in the T_2 weighted image, are present in the left cerebral hemisphere and right occipital lobe. Signal void areas corresponding to the internal carotid and main intracranial arteries are not visualized. A few signal void spots representing moyamoya vessels are seen in the right basal ganglia. Poor contrast of white and gray matter may be due to a developmental disturbance of the brain caused by cerebral ischemia which is present in this disease.

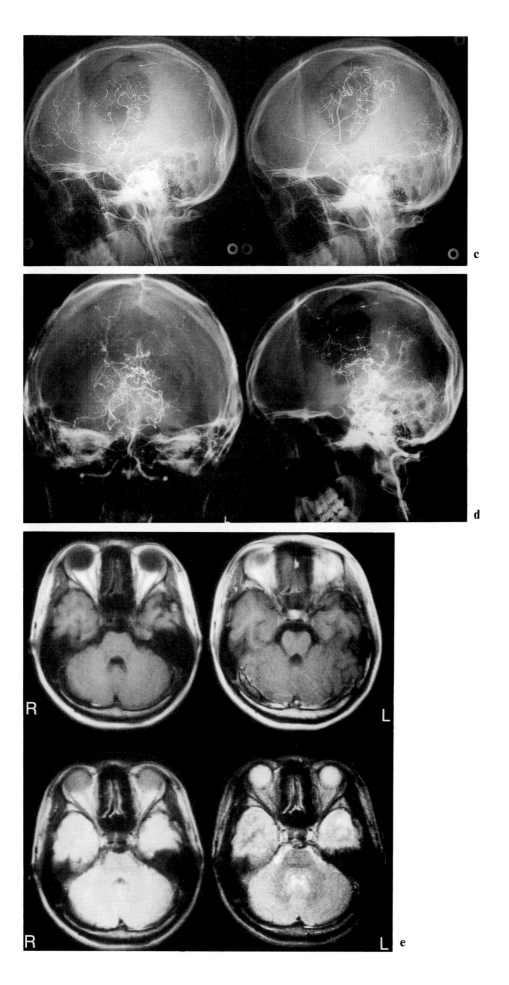

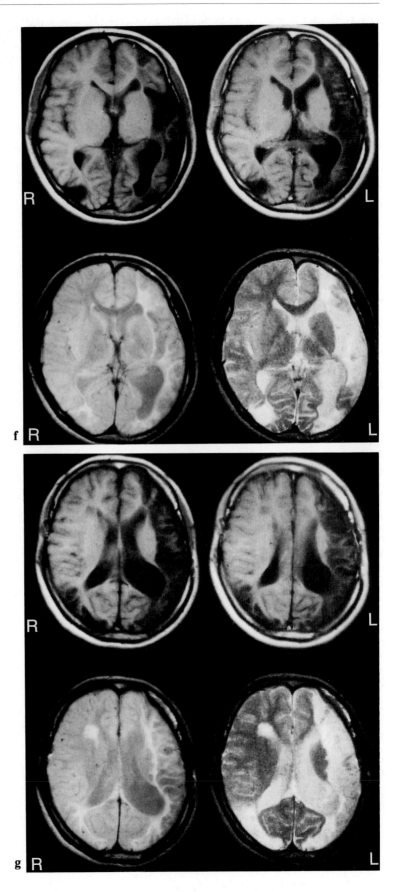

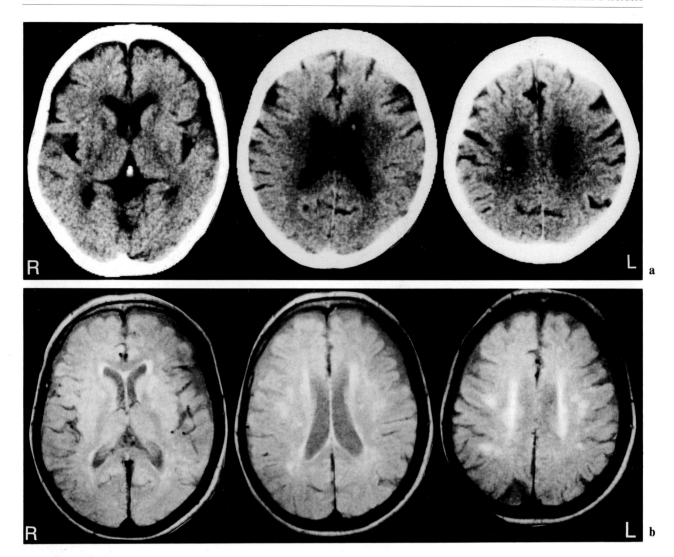

Fig. 7.14. Multiple Cerebral Infarcts. A 72-year-old female. The patient presented at our clinic after 10 days of dizziness, headache, disturbance in gait and dysarthria. Her blood pressure was 140/70 mmHg.

a *CT scan.* A plain CT revealed cerebral atrophy and a low density area in the head of the right caudate nucleus which was suspected to be a lacuna.

b *MRI.* There are multiple high signal intensity areas in both basal ganglia and extending from the corona radiata to the centrum semiovale. More infarcts are revealed on MRI than on CT. MRI is also superior to CT in the detection of cerebral ischemic changes. It can demonstrate a cerebral infarct within hours of an attack. In addition, infarcts that hitherto were not found on CT can be demonstrated by MRI.

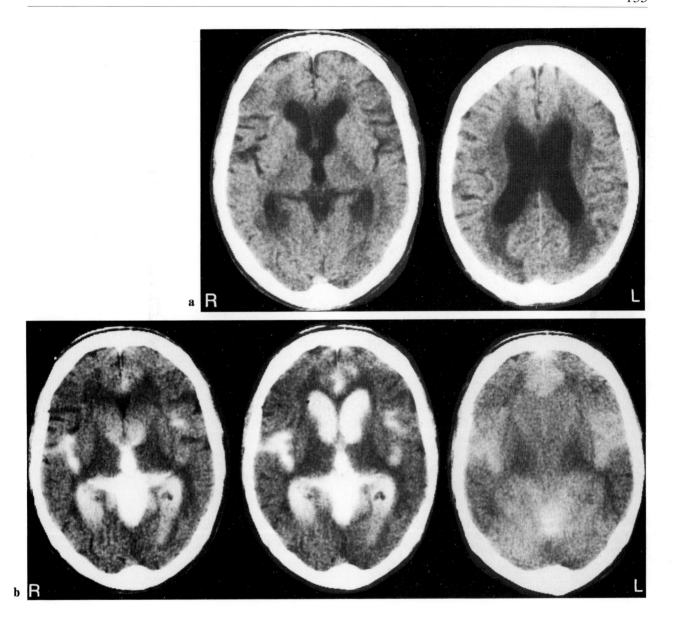

Fig. 7.15. Normal Pressure Hydrocephalus. A 62-year-old man. The patient came to our clinic with complaints of disturbances of gait, urinary incontinence and dementia.

a *CT scan.* A slight ventricular dilatation with periventricular lucency (PVL) are revealed.

b *Metrizamide CT cisternography.* Ventricular reflux and stasis are present: *left*, for 3 h; *middle*, for 6 h; *right*, for 24 h after injection of metrizamide.

c, d *MRI.* A periventricular high signal intensity (PVHI) and a high signal intensity in the basal ganglia can be seen in the T_2 weighted image. The sagittal image shows thinning of the corpus callosum. Signal void of the aqueduct is not visualized in this particular case. A diagnosis of normal pressure hydrocephalus (NPH) was made based on the clinical and radiological findings.

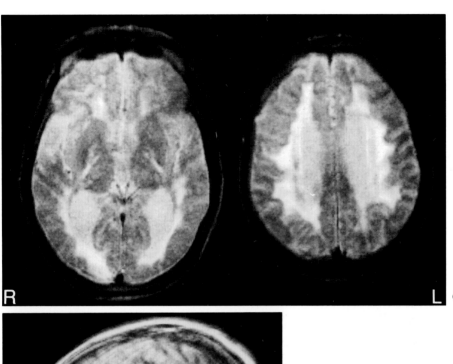

c

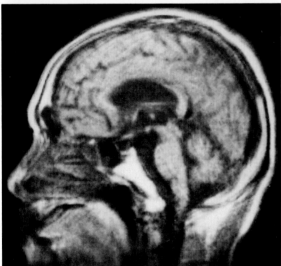

d

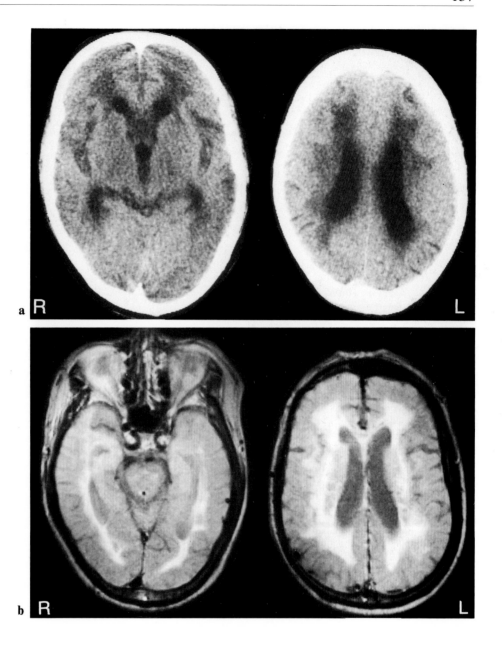

Fig. 7.16. Normal Pressure Hydrocephalus. A 73-year-old male. We were consulted because of the patient's recent development of memory disturbance and a gradually deteriorating gait.

a *CT scan.* There is a slight ventricular enlargement with periventricular lucency (PVL).

b *MRI.* A diffuse periventricular high signal intensity (PVHI) and high signal intensity spots in the white matter are seen. The aqueduct shows a signal void which is possibly due to active pulsation of the cerebrospinal fluid.

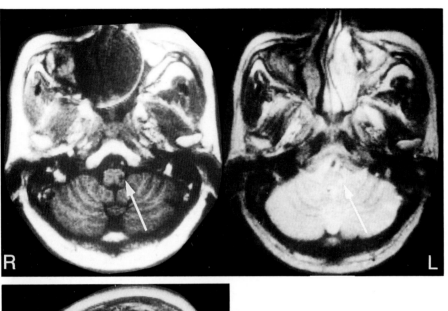

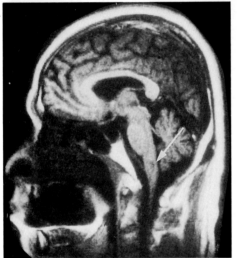

Fig. 7.17. Wallenberg's Syndrome. A 51-year-old male. The patient presented with a history of a sudden onset of dizziness and disturbances in gait. Pertinent neurological findings included: disturbance of pain and temperature sensation in the left half of the face as well as on the right half of the body, left Horner's syndrome, left cerebellar ataxia, vertigo, and hoarseness. The diagnosis was Wallenberg's syndrome.

a, b *MRI.* The T_1 weighted image shows a low signal intensity spot in the dorso-lateral part of the medulla (arrow). The T_2 image shows a high signal intensity spot in the same area (arrow). Combined with the sagittal image, a three-dimensional location of the lesion (arrow) can be determined. Due to the presence of bony artifact, it is often difficult to detect lesions in the posterior fossa. This case illustrates the usefulness of MRI in brainstem lesions.

Bibliography

Alvarez O, Hyman RA (1986) Even echo MR rephasing in the diagnosis of giant intracranial aneurysm. JCAT 10: 699–701

Alvarez O, Edwards JH, Hyman RA (1986) MR recognition of internal carotid artery occlusion. AJNR 7: 359–360

Anderson SC, Shah CP, Murtagh FR (1987) Congested deep subcortical veins as a sign of dural venous thrombosis: MR and CT correlations. JCAT 11: 1059–1061

Akiguchi H, Nabatame H, Kameyama M (1987) MRI of brainstem vascular lesions. Internal Medicine 60:857–865 (Japanese)

Aoki S (1987)) Cerebrovascular disease and MRI diagnosis. Neurological Surgery 15:589–596 (English abstract)

Atlas SW, Grossman RI, Goldberg HI, Hackney DB, Bilaniuk LT, Zimmerman RA (1987) Partially thrombosed giant intracranial aneurysms: correlation of MRI and pathologic findings. Radiology 161: 111–114

Augustyn GT, Scott JA, Olson E, Gilmor RL, Edward MK (1985) Cerebral venous angiomas: MR imaging. Radiology 156: 391–395

Biller J, Adams HP, Dunn V, Simmons Z, Jacoby CG (1986) Dichotomy between clinical findings and MR abnormalities in pontine infarction. JCAT 10: 379–385

Biller J, Yuh WTC, Mitchell GW, Bruno A, Adams HP Jr (1988) Early diagnosis of basilar artery occlusion using magnetic resonance imaging. Stroke 19: 397–306

Borello JA, Aisen AM, Gebarski SS (1986) Comparisons of MR relaxation times and X-ray attenuation coefficients in focal brain lesions. JCAT 9: 1062–1064

Bottomley PA, Drayer BP, Smith LS (1986) Chronic adult cerebral infarction studied by phosphorus NMR spectroscopy. Radiology 160: 763–766

Bradley WG, Schmidt PG (1985) Effect of methemoglobin formation on the MR appearance of subarachnoid hemorrhage. Radiology 156: 99–103

Brant-Zawadzki M, Pereira B, Weinstein P, Moore S, Kucharczyk W, Berry I, McNamara M, Derugin N (1986) MR imaging of acute experimental ischemia in cats. AJNR 7: 7–11

Brant-Zawadzki M, Weinstein P, Bartkowski H, Moseley M (1987) MR imaging and spectroscopy in clinical and experimental ischemia: a review. AJNR 8: 39–48

Braun IF, Hoffman JC, Malko JA, Pettigrew RI, Dannels W, Davis PC (1985) Jugular venous thrombosis: MR imaging. Radiology 157: 357–360

Brown JJ, Hesselink JR, Rothrock JF (1988) MR and CT of lacunar infarcts. AJNR 9: 477–482

Buonanno FS, Pykett IL, Brady TJ, Vielma J, Burt CT, Goldman MR, Hinshaw WS, Pohost GM, Kistler JP (1983) Proton NMR imaging in experimental ischemic infarction. Stroke 14: 178–184

Cammarata C, Han JS, Haaga JR, Alfidi RJ, Kaufman B (1985) Cerebral venous angiomas imaged by MR. Radiology 55: 639–643

Chakeres DW, Bryan RN (1986) Acute subarachnoid hemorrhage: in vitro comparison of magnetic resonance and computed tomography. AJNR 7: 223–228

Daniels DL, Kneeland JB, Foleyy WD, Jesmanowicz A, Froncisz W, Hyde JS (1986) Cardiac gated local coil MR imaging of the carotid bifurcation. AJNR 7: 1036–1037

Daniels DL, Pech P, Mark L, Pojunas K, Williams AL, Haughton VM (1985) Magnetic resonance imaging of the cavernous sinus. AJR 144: 1009–1014

DeLaPaz RL, New PFJ, Buonanno FS, Kistler JP, Oot RF, Rosen BR, Taveras JM, Brady TJ (1984) NMR imaging of intracranial hemorrhage. JCAT 8: 599–607

DeWitt LD, Kistler JP, Miller DC, Richardson EP Jr, Buonanno FS (1987) NMR-Neuropathologic correlation in stroke. Stroke 18: 342–851

Di Chiro G, Brooks RA, Girton ME, Caporale T, Wright DC, Dwyer AJ, Horne MK III (1986) Sequential MR studies of intracerebral hematomas in monkeys. AJNR 7: 193–199

Dooms GC, Uske A, Brant-Zawadzki M, Kucharczyk W, Lemme-Plaghos L, Newton TH, Norman D (1986) Spin-echo MR imaging of intracranial hemorrhage. Neuroradiology 28: 132–138

Dumoulin CL, Hart HR (1986) Magnetic resonance angiography. Radiology 161: 717–720

Edelman RR, Johnson K, Buxton R, Shoukimas G, Rosen BR, Davis KR, Brady TJ (1986) MR of hemorrhage: a new approach. AJNR 7: 751–756

El Gammal T, Adams RJ, Nichols FT, McKie K, Brooks BS (1986) MR and CT investigation of cerebrovascular disease in sickle cell patients. AJNR 7: 1043–1049

Fox AJ, Bogousslavsky J, Carey LS, Barnett HJM, Viniski S, Karlik SJ, Vinuela F, Pelz DM, Hachinski V (1986) Magnetic resonance imaging of small medullary infarctions. AJNR 7: 229–233

Fujisawa I, Asato R, Nishimura K, Togashi K, Itoh K, Nakano Y, Itoh H, Hashimoto N, Takeuchi J, Torizuka K (1987) Moyamoya disease. MR imaging. Radiology 164: 103–105

Goldberg HI, Grossman RI, Gomori JM, Asbury AK, Bilaniuk LT, Zimmerman RA (1986) Cervical internal carotid artery dissecting hemorrhage: diagnosis using MR. Radiology 158: 157–161

Gomori JM, Grossman RI, Goldberg HI (1985) Intracranial hematomas: imaging by high-field MR. Radiology 157: 87–93

Gomori JM, Grossman RI, Goldberg HI, Hackney DB, Zimmerman RA, Bilaniuk LT (1986) Occult cerebral vascular malformations: high field MR imaging. Radiology 158: 707–713

Gomori JM, Grossman RI, Hackney DB, Goldberg H, Zimmerman RA, Bilaniuk LT (1987) Variable appearance of subacute intracranial hematomas on high-field spin-echo MR. AJNR 8: 1019–1026

Griffin C, DeLaPaz R, Enzmann D (1987) Magnetic resonance appearance of slow flow vascular malformations of the brainstem. Neuroradiology 29: 506–511

Grossman RI, Joseph PM, Wolf G, Biery D, McGranth J, Kundel HL, Fishman JE, Zimmerman RA, Goldberg HI, Bilaniuk LT (1985) Experimental intracranial septic infarction: magnetic resonance enhancement. Radiology 155: 649–653

Hachney DB, Lesnick JE, Zimmerman RA, Grossman RI, Goldberg HI, Bilaniuk LT (1986) MR identification of bleeding site in subarachnoid hermorrhage with multiple intracranial aneurysms. JCAT 10: 878–880

Han JS, Haaga JR, Alfidi RJ, Kaufman B (1986) Cerebral venous angiomas imaged by MR. Radiology 155: 639–643

Hershey LA, Modic MT, Greenough PG, Jaffe DF, Greenough DG (1987) Magnetic resonance imaging in vascular dementia. Neurology 37: 29–36

Hirose G. Yoshioka A, Ito M, Oda R. Kataoka S (1987) Magnetic resonance imaging (MRI) in patients with acute cerebral infarction. Clin Neurol 27: 563–568 (English abstract)

Hollandd BA, Kucharczyk W, Brant-Zawadzki M, Norman D, Haas DK, Harper PS (1985) MR imaging of calcified intracranial lesions. Radiology 157: 353–356

Inao S, Furuse M, Saso K, Yoshida K, Motegi Y, Kaneoke Y, Kamata N, Izawa A (1986) Time course of NMR images and T_1 values associated with hypertensive intracerebral hematoma. Brain and Nerve 38:661–667 (English abstract)

Inoue Y, Takemoto K (1988) Cerebral hemorrhage and other vascular lesions. Journal of Medical Imagings 8:398–404 (Japanese)

Kean DM, Worthington BS, Firth JL, Hawkes RC (1987) The effects of magnetic resonance imaging on different types of microsurgical clips. J Neurol Neurosurg Psychiat 48: 286–287

Kirkpatrick JB, Hayman LA (1987) White-matter lesions in MR ranging of clinically healthy brains of elderly subjects: possible pathologic basis. Radiology 162: 509–511

Kistler JP, Buonanno FS, De Witt LD, Davis KR, Brady TJ, Fisher CM (1984) Vertebral-basilar posterior cerebral territory stroke-delineation by proton nuclear magnetic resonance imaging. Stroke 15: 417–426

Komiyama M, Baba M, Hakuba A, Nishimura S, Ioue Y (1988) MR imaging of brainstem hemorrhage. AJNR 9: 261–268

Kucharczyk W, Kelly WM, Davis DO, Norman D, Newton TH (1986) Intracranial lesions: flow-related enhancement on MR images using time-of-flight effects. Radiology 161: 767–772

Kucharczyk W, Lemme-Pleghos L, Uske A, Brant-Zawadzki M, Dooms G, Norman D (1985) Intracranial vascular lesions: MR and CT imaging. Radiology 156: 383–389

Kwan ESK, Wolpert SM, Scott RM, Runge V (1988) MR evaluation of neurovascular lesions after endovascular occlusion with detachable balloons. AJNR 9: 523–531

Leblanc RMSc, Levesque M, Comair Y, Ethier R (1987) Magnetic resonance imaging of cerebral arteriovenous malformations. Neurosurgery 21: 15–20

Lee BCP, Herzberg L, Zimmerman RD, Deck MDF (1985) MR imaging of cerebral vascular malformations. AJNR 6: 863–870

Lemme-Plaghos L, Kucharczyk W, Brant-Zawadzki M, Uske A, Edwards M, Norman D, Newton TH (1986) MR imaging of angiographically occult vascular malformations. AJNR 7: 217–222

Leonard TJK, Moseley IF, Sanders MD (1984) Ophthalmoplegia in carotid cavernous fistula. Br J Opthalmol 68: 128–134

Macchi PJ, Grossman RI, Gomori JM, Goldberg HI, Zimmerman RA, Bilaniuk LT (1986) High field MR imaging of cerebral venous thrombosis. JCAT 10: 10–15

McMurdo SK, Brant-Zawadzki M, Bradley WG, Chang GY, Berg BO (1986) Dural sinus thrombosis: study using intermediate field strength MR imaging. Radiology 161: 83–86

Naseem M, Leehey P, Russell E, Sarwar M, Devasthali R (1988) MR of basilar artery dolichoectasia. AJNR 9: 391–392

New PFJ, Ojemann RG, Davis KR, Rosen BR, Heros R, Kjelberg RN, Adams RD, Richardson EP (1988) MR and CT of occult vascular malformations of the brain. AJNR 7: 771–779

Okada A, Fujimoto T, Uetsuhara K, Asakura T, Osame M, Igata A (1987) A study of diaschisis in CVD using MR-CT. Progress in Computerized Tomography 9: 35–39 (English abstract)

Oku T, Yonemitsu T, Fujiwara S, Yoshimoto T, Suzuki J (1987) Report of a successfully operated cavernous angioma in the dorsal part of the pons: the usefulness of MRI in diagnosis. Neurological Surgery 15:159–164 (English abstract)

Rapoport S, Sostman HD, Pope C, Camputaro CM, Holcomb W, Gore JC (1987) Venous clots: evaluation with MR imaging. Radiology 162: 527–530

Rigamonti D, Drayer BP, Johnson PC, Hadley MN, Zabramski J, Spetzler RF (1987) The MRI appearance of cavernous malformations (angiomas). J Neurosurg 67: 518–524

Ruff RL, Wiener SN, Leigh RJ (1986) Magnetic resonance imaging in patients with diplopia. Invest Radiol 21: 311–319

Salgado ED, Weinstein M, Furlan AJ, Modic MT, Beck GJ, Estes M, Awad I, Little JR (1986) Proton magnetic resonance imaging in ischemic cerebrovascular disease. Ann Neurol 20: 502–507

Savino PJ, Grossman RI, Schatz NJ, Sergott RC, Bosley TM (1986) High-field magnetic resonance imaging in diagnosis of cavernous sinus thrombosis. Arch Neurol 43: 1081–1082

Schorner W, Bradac GB, Treisch J, Bender A, Felix R (1986) Magnetic resonance imaging (MRI) in the diagnosis of cerebral arteriovenous angiomas. Neuroradiology 28: 313–318

Scott JA, Augustyn GT, Gilmor RL, Mealey J Jr, Olson EW (1985) Magnetic resonance imaging of a venous angioma. AJNR 6: 284–286

Simmons Z, Biller J, Adams HP, Dunn V, Jacoby CG (1986) Cerebellar infarction: comparison of computed tomography and magnetic resonance imaging. Ann Neurol 19: 291–293

Sipponen JT (1984) Visualization of brain infarction with nuclear magnetic resonance. Neuroradiology 26: 387–391

Sipponen JT, Sepponen RE, Tanttu JI, Sivula A (1985) Intracranial hematomas studied by MR imaging at 0.17 and 0.02 T. JCAT 9: 698–704

Smith HJ, Strother CM, Kikuchi Y, Duff T, Ramirez L, Merless A, Toutant S (1988) MR imaging in the management of supratentorial intracranial AVMs. AJNR 9: 225–235

Todoroki K, Asakura T, Uetsuhara K, Kadota K, Komasaku R, Kanemaru R, Fujimoto T, Yamamoto K (1987) Magnetic resonance imaging of intracranial hematoma. Progress in Computerized Tomography 9:697–702 (English abstract)

Tsuruda JS, Halbach VV, Higasida RT, Mark AS, Hieshima GB, Norman D (1988) MR evaluation of large intracranial aneurysms using cine low flip angle gradientt-refocused imanging. AJNR 9: 415–424

Virapongse C, Mancuso A, Quisling R (1986) Human brain infarcts: Gd-DTPA enhanced MR imaging. Radiology 161: 785–794

Waluch V, Bradley WG (1984) NMR even echo rephasing in slow laminar flow. JCAT 8: 594–598

Yoon HC, Lufkin RB, Vinuela F, Bentson J, Martin N, Wilson G (1988) MR of acute subarachnoid hemorrhage. AJNR 9: 404–405

Yoshikawa K, Iio M (1986) MRI diagnosis of vascular lesions. Journal of Medical Imagings 6:1245–1252 (Japanese)

Zabramski JM, Spetzler RF, Kaufman B (1985) Magnetic resonance imaging: comparative study of radiofrequency pulse techniques in the evaluation of focal cerebral ischemia. Neurosurgery 16: 502–510

Zimmerman RD, Fleming CA, Lee BCP, Saint-Louis LA, Deck MDF (1986) Periventricular hyperintensity as seen by magnetic resonance: prevalence and significance. ANJR 7: 13–20

8 Head Injuries

There has been remarkable improvement in the ease of diagnosis of head injuries following the introduction of MRI. This includes the discovery of lesions which previously could often not be detected by CT, such as slight cerebral contusions which appear as high signal intensities in the T_2 weighted image.

The MRI diagnosis of a hemorrhage in the subacute and chronic stages is superior to that of CT, but hemorrhage in the acute stage is shown only as a low signal intensity on T_2. Care should therefore be taken not to miss subarachnoid hemorrhages, brain contusions and other similar lesions in acute stages. Subdural hematomas after the subacute phase are best demonstrated on MRI, especially the small hematomas not demonstrable by CT. Extracerebral hematomas at the base of the brain are quite difficult to detect on a CT scan.

On the other hand, in acute severe head injuries where the patient is uncooperative or connected to an artificial life support apparatus, it may not be possible to perform MRI. Its use in emergency management is therefore limited. Although the application of fast scanning techniques is expected to solve such problems, at present CT is preferred in scanning acute severe head injury cases. Despite these limitations, MRI can supplement CT: when findings compatible with clinical features cannot be obtained on CT, such as extensive shearing of the corpus callosum, they can be detected by MRI.

Detection of lesions during the subacute and chronic stages of head injuries is much better by MRI, and this should be performed initially in such cases whenever possible. Changes in brain water content in the subacute phase are especially clear in MR. Simultaneous multiplanar imaging is also possible and, since there are no bony artifacts, the lesions are well demonstrated. The detection of a shearing injury is easier by MRI than CT, but it may be difficult to differentiate a white matter lesion from primary demyelination diseases and disorders of aging. Since MRI is not usually performed in acute head injuries only a few examples of such cases are presented in this book.

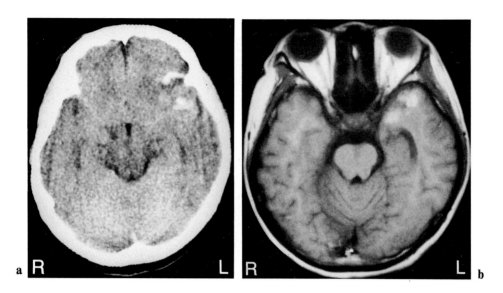

Fig. 8.1. Brain Contusion. A 21-year-old female. The patient was brought to the hospital after a traffic accident; she had a convulsive seizure upon arrival. Upon admission, the level of consciousness was 100–200 (Japan Coma Scale). Light reaction was sluggish and there was right hemiparesis.

a *CT scan.* There is a contusion in the left temporal lobe as well as subarachnoid hemorrhage.

b, c *MRI* (16 days after the accident). A patchy lesion is seen in the left temporal tip which appears with a moderately high intensity in the T_1 weighted image and a markedly high intensity in the T_2 weighted image. The morphological changes are fairly similar in both the T_1 and T_2 weighted images, and the small differences between the images may be due to the addition of slight bleeding as well as necrotic changes.

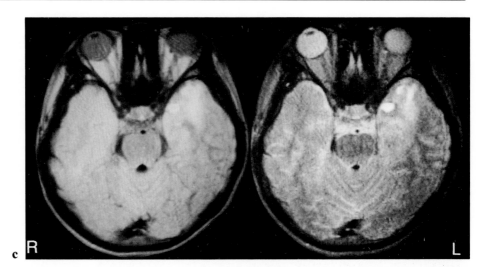

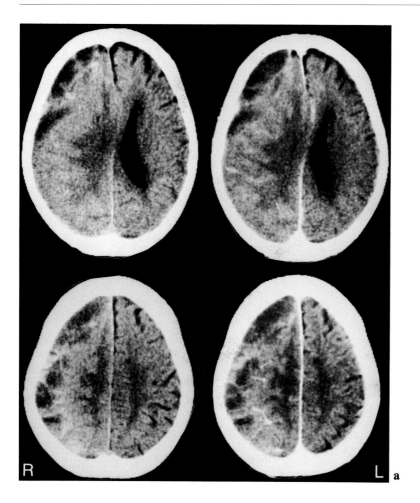

Fig. 8.2. Chronic Subdural Hematoma. A 93-year-old female. The patient developed left hemiparesis 2 weeks prior to consultation. The condition deteriorated rapidly until she became confined to bed 4 days before admission to the hospital. There was no history of head injury. Upon examination, consciousness was found to be disturbed and there was a left hemiparesis with exaggeration of deep tendon reflexes. Anisocoria was absent.

a *CT Scan.* A crescent area in the right frontoparietal region containing a mixture of low, iso, and high densities is seen. There is mass effect with collapse of the right lateral ventricle and a shift of midline structures to the left. The image of the hematoma capsule is slightly enhanced following an injection of contrast medium.

b *MRI.* The hematoma is seen as a circumscribed mass with a high signal intensity in both the T_1 and T_2 weighted images. As illustrated by this case, chronic subdural hematoma is usually seen as a high signal intensity on MRI. This may represent the signal intensity of methemoglobin. In approximately 30% of chronic subdural hematomas, the lesion may be revealed as iso to low intensity with the low density in CT corresponding to a long T_1 and the high density corresponding to a short T_1.

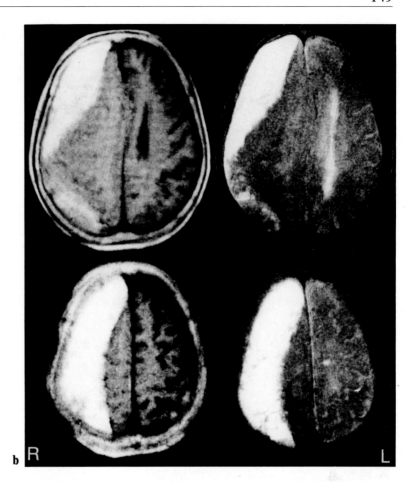

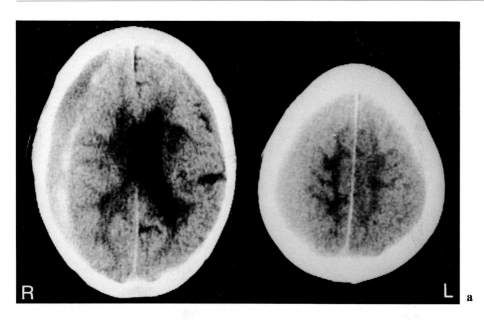

Fig. 8.3. Chronic Subdural Hematoma. A 70-year-old male. The patient fell down from a height of about 30 cm and struck his head on a hard surface 2 months prior to consultation. One month later, he was observed to have become less active and had developed a staggering gait. Upon examination, he was found to be slightly disoriented and had speech disturbance and urinary incontinence.

a *CT scan.* A crescent-shaped iso to high density area is seen in the subdural space bilaterally. The right ventricle is collapsed.

b–e *MRI.* In both T_1 and T_2 weighted images, the hematoma is shown as high signal intensity. The boundary between the brain and the hematoma is clearly defined. A diagnosis of chronic subdural hematoma was made, and irrigation was carried out through burr holes. The hematoma fluid was dark red in color and 135 ml was obtained from the right side and 45 ml from the left.

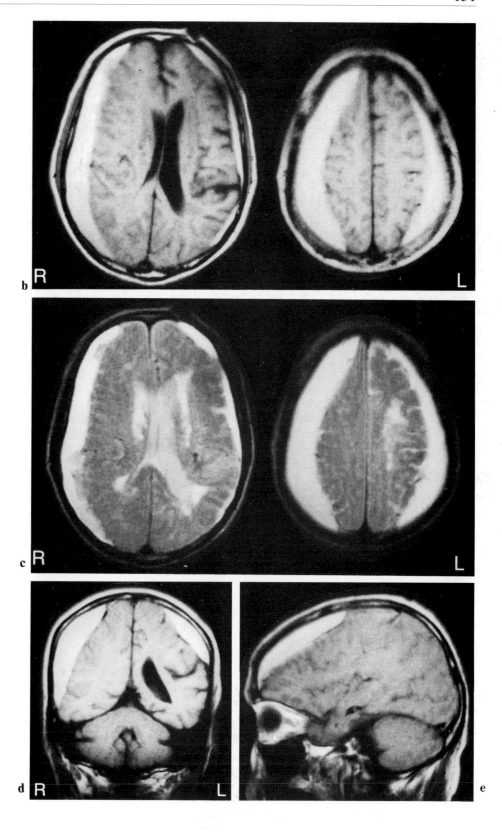

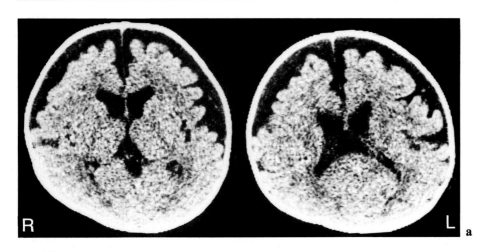

Fig. 8.4. Subdural Fluid Collection in Infancy. A 4-month-old male. The baby was delivered normally after a normal full-term pregnancy. The postnatal period was uneventful. At a routine 4 month check-up, the anterior fontanelle was noticed to be bulging and he exhibited the sunset phenomenon.

a *CT scan.* A low density area is seen extending over both frontal lobes and the cerebral sulci are clearly demonstrated. There is no hydrocephalus.

b–e *MRI.* In the T_1 weighted image, a low signal intensity is seen in the same area as the lesion revealed on CT; however, it appears as a high signal intensity in the T_2 weighted image. These findings are compatible with the presence of CSF. A diagnosis of subdural effusion was made from the CT and MRI findings.

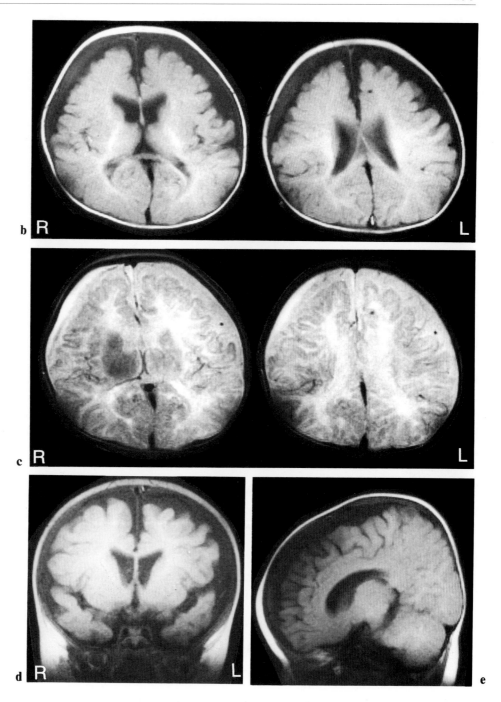

Bibliography

DeLaPas RL, New PFJ, Buonanno FS, Kistler JP, Oot RF, Rosen BR, Taveras JM, Brady TJ (1984) MR imaging of intracranial hemorrhage. JCAT 8: 599–607

Gentry LR, Godersky JC, Thompson B (1988) MR imaging of head trauma: review of the distribution and radiopathologic features of traumatic lesions. AJNR 9: 101–110

Gentry LR Godersky JC, Thompson B, Dunn VD (1988) Prospective comparative study of intermediate-field MR and CT in the evaluation of closed head trauma. AJNR 9: 91–100

Gomori JM, Grossman RI, Goldberg HI, Zimmerman RA, Bilaniuk LT (1985) Intracranial hematomas; imaging by high-field MR. Radiology 157: 87–93

Gomori JM, Grossman RI, Hackney DB, Goldberg HI, Zimmerman RA, Bilaniuk LT (1987) Variable appearances of subacute intracranial hematomas on high-field spin-echo MR. AJNR 8: 1019-1026, Radiology 157: 87–93

Hans JS, Huss RG, Benson JE, Kaufman B, Yoon YS, Morrison SC, Alfidi RJ, Rekate HL, Ratcheson RA (1984) MR imaging of the skull base. JCAT 8: 944–952

Han JS, Kaufman B, Alfidi RJ, Yeung HN, Benson JE, Haaga JR, EI Yousef SJ, Clampitt ME, Bonstelle CT, Huss R (1984) Head trauma evaluated by magnetic resonance and computed tomography: a comparison. Radiology 150: 71–77

Hesselink JR, Dowd CF, Healy ME, Hajek P, Baker LL, Luerssen TG (1988) MR imaging of brain contusions: a comparative study with CT. AJNR 9: 269–278

Inao S, Furuse M, Saso K, Yoshida K, Motegi Y, Kaneoke Y, Izawa A (1987) Significance of focal relaxation times in head injury. Neurol Med Chir 27:10-39–1045 (English abstract)

Jenkins A, Teasdale G, Hadley MDM, Macpherson P, Rowan JO (1986) Brain lesions detected by magnetic resonance imaging in mild and severe head injuries. Lancet 2: 445–446

Kelly AB, Zimmerman RD, Snow RB, Gandy SE, Heier LA, Deck MDF (1988) Head trauma: comparison of MR and CT-experience in 100 patients. AJNR 9: 699–708

Langfitt TW, Obrist WD, Alavi A, Grossman RI, Zimmerman R, Jaggi J, Lizzell B, Reivich M, Patton DR (1986) Computerized tomography, magnetic resonance imaging and positron emission tomography in the study of brain trauma. J Neurosurg 64: 760–767

Levin HS, Handel SF, Goldman AM, Eisenberg HM, Guinto FC Jr (1985) Magnetic resonance imaging after 'diffuse' nonmissile head injury. Arch Neurol 42: 963–968

Moon KL Jr, Brant-Zawadzki M, Pitts LH, Millls CM (1984) Nuclear magnetic resonance imaging of CT-isodense subdural hematomas. AJNR 5: 319–322

Sipponen JT, Sepponen RE, Sivula A (1984) Chronic subdural hematoma: demonstration by magnetic resonance. Radiology 150: 79–85

Sipponen JT, Sepponen RE, Tanttu JI, Silvula A (1985) Intracranial hematomas studied by MR imaging at 0.17 and 0.02 T. JCAT 9: 698–704

Yamada K, Matsuzawa T, Yamada S, Yoshioka S, Ono S (1986) Magnetic resonance imaging and relaxation time studies of brain oedema. Adv Neurol Sci 30: 451–460 (English abstract)

Zimmerman RA, Bilaniuk LT, Grossman RI, Levine RS, Lynch R, Goldberg HI, Samuel L, Edelstein W, Bottomley P, Redington RW (1985) Resistive NMR of intracranial hematomas. Neuroradiology 27: 16–20

Zimmerman RA, Bilaniuk LT, Hachney DB, Goldberg HI, Grossman RI (1986) Head injury: early results of comparing CT and high-field MR. AJNR 7: 757–764

9 Congenital Anomalies and Pediatric Diseases

Congenital anomalies of the central nervous system are defined as anomalies present at birth. Most cause difficulties during childhood and constitute a large proportion of pediatric neurological disorders.

Malformations have characteristic morphological changes, making it possible to diagnose most of them by CT scans and MRIs. The structural anatomy of both the brain and spinal cord is superbly demonstrated on MRI by the T_1 weighted image. The T_2 weighted image is useful in the diagnosis of both congenital tumors and tumors seen in neurocutaneous syndromes, as well as in investigating the properties of fluid collection. In most cases, the T_1 weighted image is the main diagnostic tool. The superiority of MRI over CT (in the diagnosis of malformations) lies in the fact it can display three-dimensional configurations of lesions including sagittal images. Posterior fossa lesions (Chiari malformations, Dandy Walker cysts and others) are well demonstrated by virtue of their relationship to the fourth ventricle and craniovertebral junction. In Chiari malformations, the diagnosis of syringomyelia is possible in the mid-sagittal section of the spinal cord.

The diagnosis of spinal dysraphism became quite easy following the introduction of MRI. Thus, lesions like syringomyelias, the tethered cord syndrome, spinal lipomas, and others, which are difficult to recognize on CT, can now be clearly demonstrated on MRI. Spinal cord tumors also can now be more easily diagnosed due to their signal intensities on both T_1 and T_2 weighting.

The dynamics of cerebrospinal fluid (CSF) in congenital hydrocephalus can be examined by CT cisternography. With the introduction of cine MRI which shows the flow clearly, it has now become possible to observe the flow of CSF. Thus, it is possible to observe the to-and-fro movements of CSF within the aqueduct, and the exit and entry of CSF into a syrinx.

In children, particularly during infancy, the pathogenesis of certain lesions such as chronic subdural fluid collections remains unclear, and diagnosis and treatment are often difficult. Due to the signal intensities of the T_1 and T_2 weighted images, MRI makes it easy to distinguish whether the fluid collection is a hematoma or CSF. It is believed that MRI will eventually contribute more to the characterization of pathologic processes in the future.

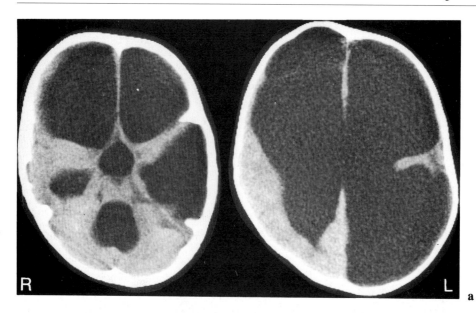

Fig. 9.1. Hydrocephalus. A 5-year-old male. The child was delivered normally after an uneventful full-term pregnancy. He developed ventricular hemorrhage at the age of 1 month and ventricular drainage was performed. However, this was complicated by purulent meningitis which was treated with antibiotics. A shunt operation was considered for the post meningitic hydrocephalus but the idea was abandoned because it was thought that the patient would be unable to tolerate the procedure. He started sitting unaided at the age of 4 years. His speech is retarded and at present he can only utter a few words at a time. He was referred to our clinic for a shunt operation.

a *CT scan.* Marked panventricular dilatation is seen.

b *MRI.* This shows the same findings as those seen on CT. The center of the fourth ventricle is shown as a low signal intensity in the T_2 weighted image. This may be related to the dynamics of CSF.

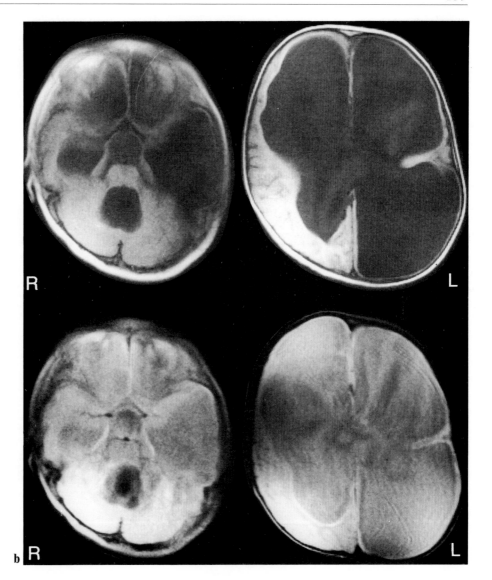

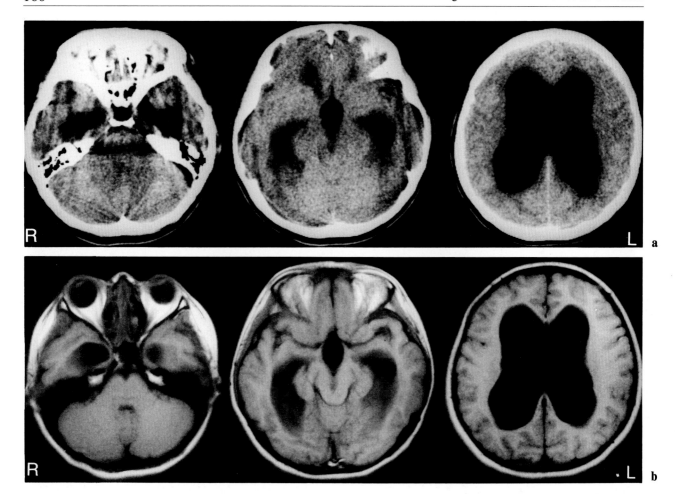

Fig. 9.2. Hydrocephalus. A 14-year-old female. The patient had an attack of headache located in the right orbital region and radiating to the parietal area. This was associated with nausea and vomiting. She consulted a physician and was given analgesics. One month before consultation, she had a repeat attack and was taken to the internal medicine department of our hospital. A CT scan was done revealing hydrocephalus and the patient was referred to our clinic for further evaluation. Upon examination, she was found to have papilledema.

a *CT scan.* There is marked dilation of the lateral and third ventricles.

b–e *MRI.* Findings similar to those of CT are observed. Narrowing of the aqueduct is visible in the sagittal image. The diagnosis of hydrocephalus due to aqueductal stenosis was made based on CT and MRI findings.

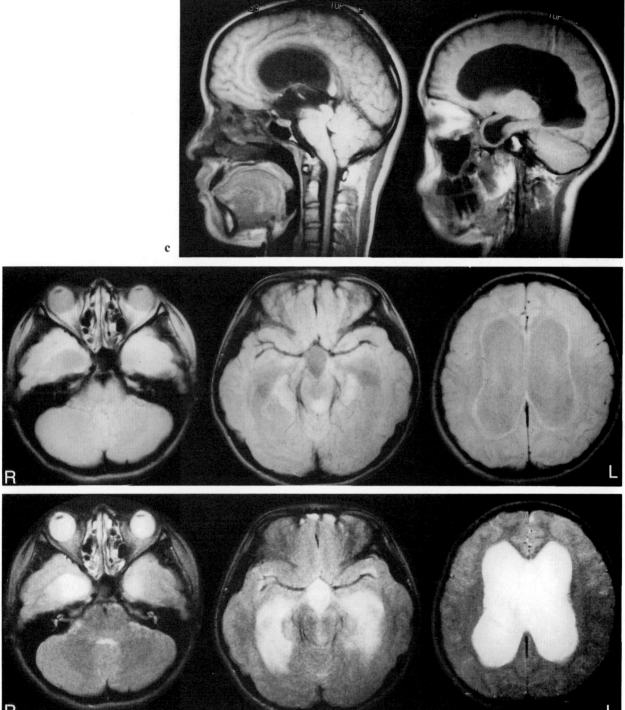

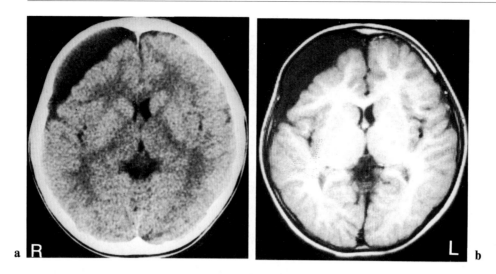

Fig. 9.3. Anterior Fossa Arachnoid Cyst. An 8-year-old male. During the previous 2 months, the patient had two episodes of headaches accompanied by vomiting. A cyst was discovered in the right frontal region by a CT scan and the child was referred to our service for admission.

a *CT scan.* A low density area with minimal mass effect is seen in the right frontal region.

b–d *MRI.* The low density area in CT is shown as a low signal intensity in the T_1 weighted image. This signal pattern is similar to that of CSF. A convexity arachnoid cyst was diagnosed from the CT and MRI findings.

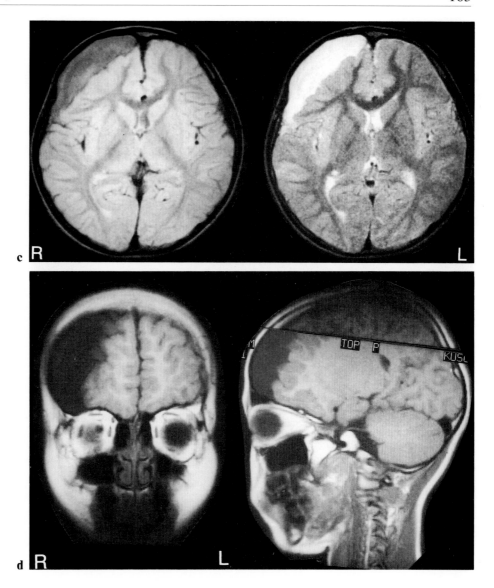

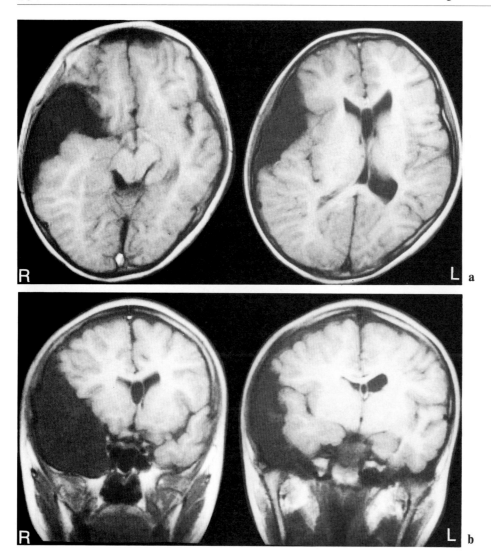

Fig. 9.4. Middle Fossa Arachnoid Cyst. A 10-year-old female. The child fell from a ladder 1 month prior to consultation. Although she suffered no injury at the time, she subsequently complained of headaches and was taken to a physician who discovered some abnormality on a CT scan. The neurological examination was negative.

a, b *MRI.* A diffuse low signal intensity area is seen in the right middle fossa in the T_1 weighted image. There is a marked mass effect with compression of the right temporal horn and adjacent areas and midline shift. There is an associated dysgenesis of the right temporal lobe and cavum septi pellucidi. From the above findings, the diagnosis of an arachnoid cyst in the right middle cranial fossa was made.

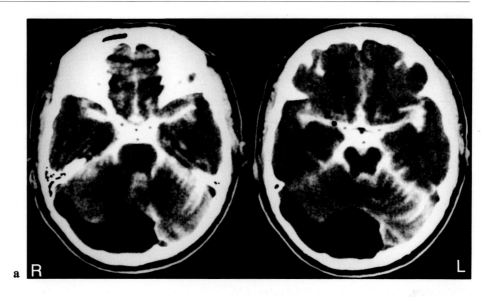

Fig. 9.5. Posterior Fossa Arachnoid Cyst. A 46-year-old female. The patient consulted a physician because of vertigo, nausea, and vomiting. A CT scan showed a cystic lesion in the posterior cranial fossa and she was referred to our clinic. Upon admission, nystagmus with a quick component to the right was observed.

a *Metrizamide cisternography.* There is no filling of the contrast medium into the cyst cavity.

b, c *MRI.* A mass is seen in the posterior fossa, appearing as a low signal intensity in the T_1 weighted image and as a high signal intensity in the T_2 weighted image. There is thinning of the occipital bone as well as mass effect on the cerebellum. The lesion was diagnosed from the CT and MRI findings as a retrocerebellar arachnoid cyst.

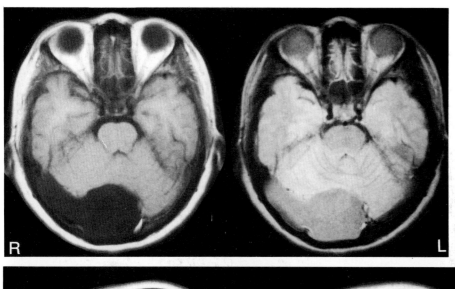

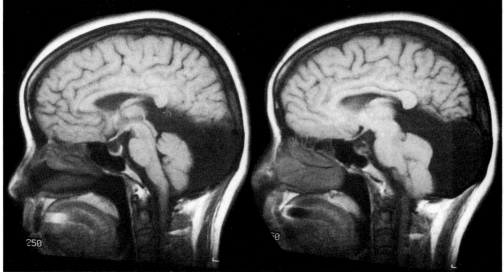

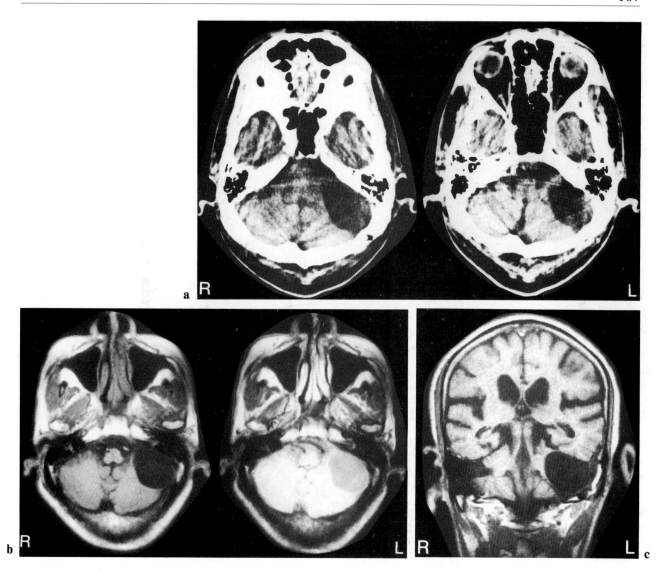

Fig. 9.6. Cerebellopontine Angle Arachnoid Cyst. A 76-year-old male. The patient presented with a 2-week history of numbness in his right hand. Upon examination, hypesthesia of the right hand and cerebellar symptoms were present.

a *CT scan.* A low density area with minimal mass effect is seen in the left cerebellopontine angle, and the injection of a contrast medium did not enhance the image.

b, c *MRI.* A low signal intensity mass in the T_1 weighted image and a high signal intensity in the T_2 weighted image is seen in the same area as noted on CT. The lesion was diagnosed as an arachnoid cyst due to the similarity between its signal intensity and that associated with CSF.

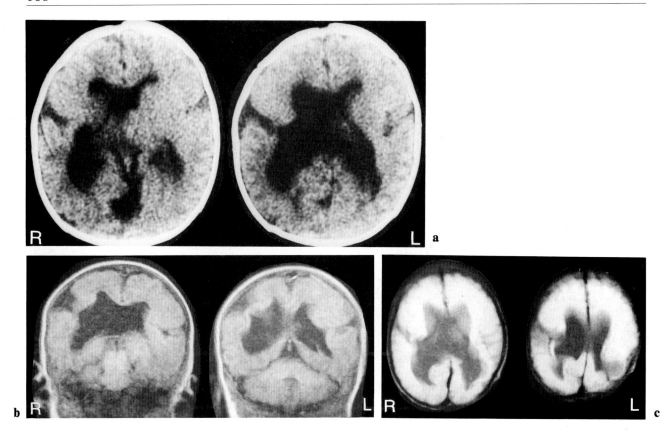

Fig. 9.7. Schizencephaly. A 1-month-old male. The pregnancy and delivery were unremarkable, and he was referred to our clinic because he was microcephalic..

a *CT scan.* There is slight ventricular dilatation and a cleft can be seen between the right lateral ventricle and the Sylvian fissure.

b, c *MRI.* The findings on MRI are almost the same as those seen on CT. The cleft is well demonstrated in the coronal image. The patient was diagnosed as having schizencephaly based on the CT and MRI findings.

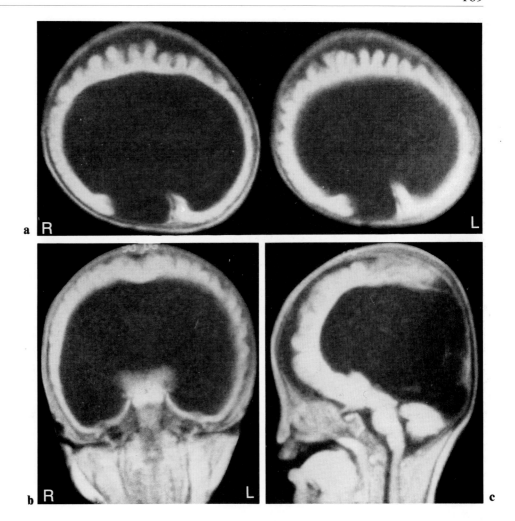

Fig. 9.8. Holoprosencephaly. A 2-year-old female. After a normal delivery, it was noted that the baby had a cleft lip and palate. A month after birth, her head circumference was around 8 cm larger than the normal size. She subsequently developed diabetes insipidus and had frequent convulsions.

a-c *MRI*. There is no visible interhemispheric fissure. The ventricle is monoventricular without formation of lateral ventricles. The fourth ventricle is normal but the third ventricle is absent. Some brain parenchyma is observed in the anterior area. The dorsal sac is connected to the monoventricle in the posterior region. From the MRI findings, the diagnosis of holoprocencephaly of the alobar type was made. (Courtesy of Dr. Sakota)

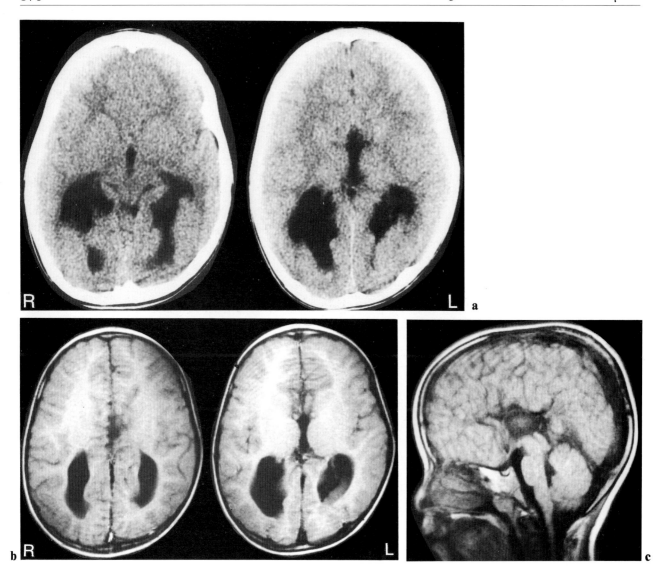

Fig. 9.9. Agenesis of the Corpus Callosum. A 5-year-old male. The child developed visual disturbances which gradually worsened several months prior to consulting an ophthalmologist. Bilateral atrophy of the optic discs was diagnosed and the patient was referred to our clinic. Other pertinent findings included psychomotor retardation.

a *CT scan.* The frontal horns of both lateral ventricles are abnormal in size and separated laterally, while both posterior horns are dilated. A third ventricle that is both dilated and elevated is insinuated between the lateral ventricles.

b, c *MRI.* Complete absence of the corpus callosum is seen in the sagittal image.

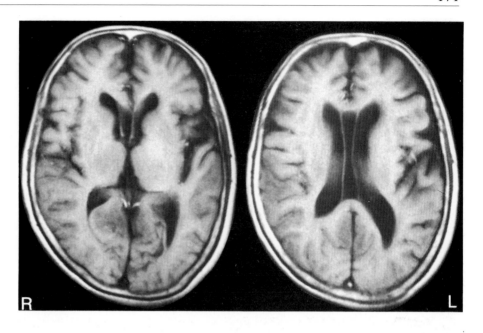

Fig. 9.10. Cavum Septi Pellucidi and Vergae. A 68-year-old female. The patient presented at our clinic with a history of fever, headaches, and slight disturbance of consciousness followed by convulsions. A neurological examination revealed nuchal rigidity. She was diagnosed as having meningitis after an examination of the CSF.

MRI. In the T_1 weighted image, a low intensity area similar to that of CSF is seen between the lateral ventricles. There is also slight cortical atrophy.

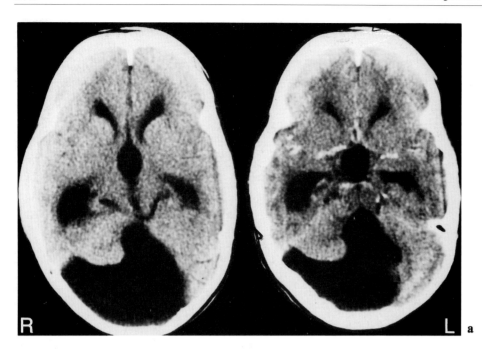

Fig. 9.11. Dandy-Walker Cyst. An 8-year-old female. The child was brought to our clinic with a history of headaches. The physical examination revealed nuchal tenderness and an ataxic gait.

a *CT scan.* A large low density area is seen in the posterior fossa, and communicates with the fourth ventricle. The cerebellar vermis is hypoplastic and the cerebellar hemispheres are separated laterally.

b *Metrizamide CT cisternography.* A CT scan evaluated 3 h after an intrathecal injection of metrizamide shows the presence of the dye in the suprasellar cistern and Sylvian fissure, but it does not pass into the cyst cavity.

c, d *MRI.* As shown on CT, the relation of the low signal intensity area in the posterior fossa to the fourth ventricle, hypoplasia of the cerebellar vermis, and hydrocephalus are well displayed.

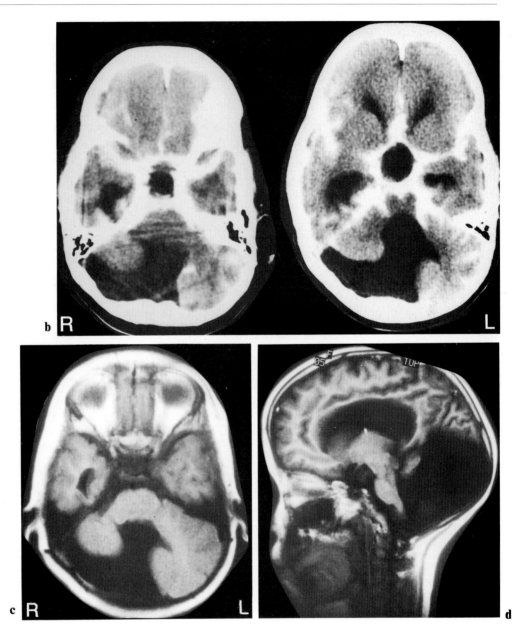

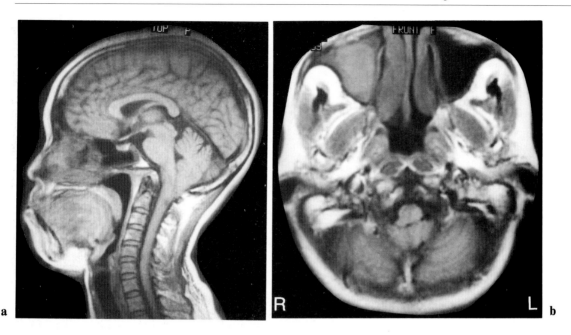

Fig. 9.12. Chiari Type 1 Malformation. A 47-year-old female. The patient noticed numbness in the left lower extremity 1 year prior to consultation. Two months ago, she experienced numbness extending from the right shoulder to the fingertips. The neurological examination revealed the presence of weakness and numbness in both right upper and lower extremities.

a, b *MRI*. In the T_1 weighted sagittal image, the cerebellar tonsils are seen to have lost the normal curvilinear configuration and have assumed a tongue-like appearance. This is compatible with findings typical of a Chiari type 1 malformation. There is associated platybasia, while syringomyelia is absent. In the T_1 weighted axial image, downward protruding semilunar cerebellar tonsils are seen behind the cord. The low intensity area in the center of the border between the spinal cord and tonsils may represent an outlet for CSF.

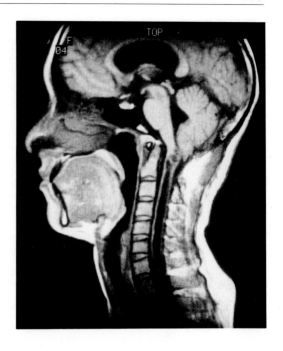

Fig. 9.13. Chiari Type 1 Malformation. A 25-year-old female. The patient had first noticed numbness of the left upper extremity 7 years ago. This had been accompanied by weakness and atrophy of the intrinsic muscles of the left hand. Following consultation at another hospital, she was informed that she had a Chiari malformation, syringomyelia, and hydrocephalus, and subsequently underwent a suboccipital decompression and ventriculo peritoneal shunt procedure.

MRI. There is downward displacement of the cerebellar tonsil and medulla into the cervical canal, and syringomyelia can be seen at the level of C_2 and below in the sagittal image.

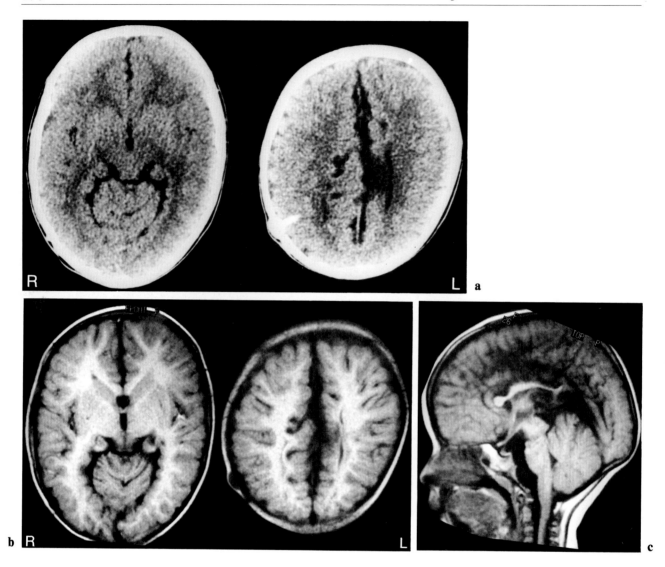

Fig. 9.14. Chiari Type 2 (Arnold-Chiari) Malformation. A 2-year-old female. Hydramnios was noted during pregnancy and the umbilical cord was twisted at delivery. The weight at birth was 3,570 gm. A myelomeningocele which was present in the lumbosacral region at birth was repaired. Two days after delivery a V-P shunt was inserted for the hydrocephalus. At present, there is weakness of the feet, pes equinovarus, and urinary and fecal incontinence. Mental development is within normal limits.

a *CT scan.* The ventricle is slit-like and the characteristic findings of a Chiari type 2 malformation, such as tectum beaking, interdigitation of the cerebral hemisphere, and hypoplasia of the tentorium, are present.

b, c *MRI.* The findings are the same as those seen on CT. In the sagittal image, downward displacement of the vermis and brainstem into the cervical canal and agenesis of the corpus callosum are also seen.

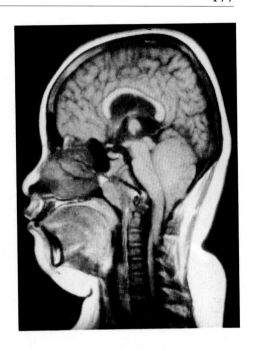

Fig. 9.15. Chiari Type 2 (Arnold-Chiari) Malformation. A 9-year-old female. The child was delivered following successful induction of labor after 10 months of gestation. A myelomeningocele and hydrocephalus were noted at birth. Immediately after delivery, repair of the hernia and the placement of a V-P shunt were performed. Upon examination, flaccid paraparesis and dislocation of the hip joint were observed.

MRI. Enlargement of the ventricle and downward displacement of the cerebellar vermis into the cervical canal are seen. Anomalies commonly associated with type 2 malformations, such as large massa intermedia, tectum beaking, upward displacement of the cerebellar vermis, and buckling of an elongated medulla over the spinal cord are present. The fourth ventricle is collapsed and there is no syringomyelia. The sagittal image is useful in demonstrating the downward displacement of the cerebellum and brainstem and the position of the fourth ventricle in relation to the foramen magnum.

Bibliography

Aboulezz AO, Sartor K, Geuer CA, Gado MH (1985) Position of the cerebellar tonsils in the normal population and in patients with Chiari malformation: a quantitative approach with MR imaging. JCAT 9: 1033–1036

Altman NR, Altman DH (1987) MR imaging of spinal dysraphism. ANJR 8: 533–538

Asano N, Oi S (1987) Cranium bifidum associated with unusual intracranial extension: MRI findings and possible pathogenesis. Neurol Med Chir 27: 1114–1119 (English abstract)

Atlas SW, Zimmerman RA, Bilaniuk LT, Rorke L, Hackney DB, Goldberg HI, Grossman RI (1986) Corpus callosum and limbic system: neuroanatomic MR evaluation of developmental anomalies. Radiology 160: 355–362

Atlas SW, Zimmerman RA, Bruce D, Schut L, Bilaniuk LT, Hackney DB (1988) Neurofibromatosis and agenesis of the corpus callosum in identical twins: MR diagnosis. AJNR 9: 598–601

Bairamian D, Di Chiro G, Theodore WH, Holmes MD, Dorwart RH, Lasson SM (1985) Case report. MR imaging and positron emission tomography of cortical heterotopia. JCAT 9: 1137–1139

Barkovich AJ, Chuang SH, Norman D (1987) MR of neuronal migration anomalies. AJNR 8: 1009–1017

Barkovich AJ, Kjos BO (1988) Normal postnatal development of the corpus callosum as demonstrated by MR imaging. AJNR 9: 487–491

Barkovich AJ, Norman D (1988a) MR imaging of schizencephaly. AJNR 9: 297–302

Barkovich AJ, Norman D (1988b) Anomalies of the corpus callosum: correlation with further anomalies of the brain. AJNR 9: 493–501

Barnes PD, Lester PD, Yamanashi WS, Prince JR (1986) Magnetic resonance imaging in infants and children with spinal dysraphism. AJNR 7: 465–472

Bergstrand G, Bergstrom M, Nordell B, Stahlberg F, Ericsson A, Hemmingeson A, Sperber G, Thuomas K-A, Jung B (1985) Cardiac gated MR imaging of cerebrospinal fluid flow. JCAT 9: 1003–1006

Bewermeyer H, Bamborschke S, Ebhardt G, Hunermann B, Heiss W-D (1985) MR imaging in adrenoleukomyeloneuropathy. JCAT 9: 793–796

Bewermeyer H, Dreesbach HA, Hunermann B, Heiss W-D (1984) MR imaging of familiar basilar impression. JCAT 8: 953–956

Bonganno JR, Edwards MK, Lee TA, Dunn DW, Roos KL, Klatte EC (1988) Cranial MR imaging in neurofibromatosis. AJNR 9: 461–468

Bosley TM, Cohen DA, Schatz NJ, Zimmerman RA, Bilaniuk LT, Savino PJ, Sergott RS (1985) Comparison of metrizamide computed tomography and magnetic resonance imaging in the evaluation of lesions at the cervicomedullary junction. Neurology 35: 485–492

Bradley WG, Kortman KE, Burgoyne B (1986) Flowing cerebrospinal fluid in normal and hydrocephalic states: appearance on MR images. Radiology 159: 611–616

Brown EW, Riccardi VM, Mawad M, Handel S, Goldman A, Bryan RN (1987) MR imaging of optic pathways in patients with neurofibromatosis. AJNR 8: 1031–1036

Condon D, Patterson J, Wyper D, Haliday D, Grant R, Teasdale G (1986) The use of magnetic resonance imaging to measure the intracranial cerebrospinal fluid volume. Lancet 1: 1355–1357

Curned JT, Laster DW, Koubek TD, Moody DM, Ball MR, Witcofski RL (1986) MRI of corpus callosal syndromes. AJNR 7: 617–622

Davidson HD, Abraham RE, Steiner RE (1985) Agenesis of the corpus callosum: magnetic resonance imaging. Radiology 155: 371–373

Deeb ZL, Rothfus WE, Maroon JC (1985) MR imaging of heterotopic gray matter. JCAT 9: 1149–1151

Dubowitz LMS, Bydder GM (1985) Nuclear magnetic resonance imaging in the diagnosis and follow-up of neonatal cerebral injury. Clin Perinatol 12: 243–260

Dubowitz LMS, Pennock JM, Johnson MA, Bydder GM (19866) High resolution magnetic resonance imaging of the brain in children. Clin Radiol 37: 113–117

Dunn V, Mock T, Bell WE, Smith W (1986) Detection of heterotopic gray matter in children by magnetic resonance imaging. Mag Res Imag 4: 33–39

El Gammal T, Allen MB Jr, Brooks BS, Mark EK (1987) MR evaluation of hydrocephalus. AJNR 8: 591–597

El Gammal T, Mark EK, Brooks BS (1987) MR imaging of Chiari II malformation. AJNR 8: 1037–1044

Han JS, Benson JE, Kaufman B, Rekate HL, Alfidi RJ, Huss RG, Sacco D, Yoon YS, Morrison SC (1985) MR imaging of pediatric cerebral abnormalities. JCAT 9: 103–114

Hanigan WC, Gibson J, Kleopoulos NJ, Cusack T, Zwicky G, Wright RM (1986) Medical imaging of fetal ventriculomegaly. J Neurosurg 64: 575–580

Harsh GR, Edwards MSB, Wilson CB (1986) Intracranial arachnoid cysts in children. J Neurosurg 64: 835–842

Hata Y, Miyamoto Y, Tada S, Kobari T (1986) Study on anomalies of the craniovertebral junction by MRI. Journal of Medical Imagings 6:625–631 (Japanese)

Hatayama R, Noguchi J (1985) Basilar impression combined with Arnold-Chiari malformation and syringobulbia: MRI (magnetic resonance image, NMR) diagnosis. Acta Soc Ophthalmol Jpn 89:654–659 (English abstract)

Inoue T, Matsushima T, Nakagaki H, Fukui M, Fukushima T, Kuromatsu C, Takagi T, Hasuo K, Koga T (1987) Magnetic resonance imaging of intracranial arachnoid cysts: with emphasis on differentiation from low-grade glioma. Nerv Syst Child 12:233–241 (English abstract)

Jocoby CG, Yuh WTC, Afifi AK, Bell WE, Schelper RL, Sato Y (1987) Accelerated myelination in early Sturge-Weber syndrome demonstrated by MR imaging. JCAT 11: 226–231

Johnson MA, Desai S, Hugh-Jones K, Starer F (1984) Magnetic resonance imaging of the brain in Hurler syndrome. AJNR 5: 816–819

Johnson MA, Pennock JM, Bydder GM, Dubowitz LMS, Thomas DJ, Young IR
    (1987) Serial MR imaging in neonatal cerebral injury. AJNR 8: 83–92
Kawamura M, Yagishita T, Kojima S, Hirayama K, Soma Y, Arimizu N (1985)
    Magnetic resonance imaging in agenesis of corpus callosum. Brain and Nerve
    37:1203–1210 (English abstract)
Kawamura M, Hirayama K (1986) Interhemispheric disconnexion syndrome due
    to callosal lesions and its diagnosis by magnetic resonance imaging. Adv
    Neurol Sci 30:461–473 (English abstract)
Kean DM, Smith MA, Douglas RHB, Martyn CN, Best JJK (1985) Two examples
    of CNS lipomas demonstrated by computed tomography and low field (0.08
    T) MR imaging. JCAT 9: 494–496
Kemp SS, Zimmerman RA, Bilaniuk LT, Hackney DB, Goldberg HI, Grossman
    RI (1987) Magnetic resonance imaging of the cerebral aqueduct. Neuro-
    radiology 29: 430–436
Kinglsey DPE, Kendall BE, Fitz CR (1986) Tuberous sclerosis: a clinicoradiological
    evaluation of 110 cases with particular reference to atypical presentation.
    Neuroradiology 28: 38–46
Kjos BO, Brant-Zawakzki M, Kucharczyk W, Kelly WM, Norman D, Newton
    TH (1985) Cystic intracranial lesions: magnetic resonance imaging. Radiology
    155: 363–369
Koch TK, Yee MHC, Hutchinson HT, Berg BO (1986) Magnetic resonance
    imaging in subacute necrotizing encephalomyelopathy (Leigh's disease). Ann
    Neurol 19: 605–607
Kykmen E, Marsh WR, Baker HL (1985) Magnetic resonance imaging in
    syringomyelia. Neurosurgery 17: 267–270
Le Bihan D, Breton E, Aubin ML, Lallemand D, Vignaud J (1987) Study of
    cerebrospinal fluid dynamics by MRI of intravoxel incoherent motions. J
    Neuroradiol 14: 388–395
Lee BC, Deck MD, Kneeland JB, Cahill PT (1985) MR imaging of the
    craniocervical junction. AJNR 6: 209–213
Lee BC, Zimmerman RD, Manning JJ, Deck MD (1985) MR imaging of
    syringomyelia and hydromyelia. AJNR 66: 221–228
Littrup JP, Gebarski SS (1985) MR imaging in Hallervorden-Spatz disease. JCAT
    9: 491–493
Martin N, Broucker T, Cambier J, Marsault C, Nahum H (1987) MRI evaluation
    of tuberous sclerosis. Neuroradiology 29: 437–443
Mayer JS, Kulkarni MV, Yeakley JW (1987) Craniocervical manifestations of
    neurofibromatosis: MR versus CT studies. JCAT 11: 839–844
McArdle CB, Nicholas DA, Richardson CJ, Amparo EG (1986) Monitoring of the
    neonate undergoing MR imaging: technical considerations. Radiology 159:
    223–226
McArdle CB, Richardson CJ, Nicholas DA, Mirfakhraee M, Hayden CK, Amparo
    EG (1987a) Developmental features of the neonatal brain: MR imaging, part 1.
    Gray-white matter differentiation and myelination. Radiology 162: 223–229
McArdle CB, Richardson CJ, Nicholas DA, Mirfakhraee M, Hayden CK, Amparo
    EG (1987b) Developmental features of the neonatal brain: MR imaging, part
    2. Ventricular size and extracerebral space. Radiology 162: 230–234

McCarthy SM, Filly RA, Stark DD, Callen PW, Golbus MS, Hricak H (1985) Magnetic resonance imaging of fetal anomalies in utero: early experience AJR 145: 677–682

McMurdo SK, Moore SG, Brant-Zawadzki M, Berg BO, Koch T, Newton TH, Edwards MSB (1987) MR imaging of intracranial tuberous sclerosis. AJNR 8: 77–82

Miller ME, Kido D, Horner F (1986) Cavum Vergae, association with neurologic abnormality and diagnosis by magnetic resonance imaging. Arch Neurol 43: 8211–823

Miyamoto Y, Hata Y, Tada S (1984) MRI investigation of syringomyelia. Journal of NMR Medicine 4:48–53 (English abstract)

Mori K (1985) Anomalies of the central nervous system. Neuroradiology and neurosurgery. Thieme-Stratton, New York

Mori K, Handa H (1987) Congenital Anomalis of the Central Nervous System. New edition. Neuron Press, Tokyo (Japanese)

Ohara S, Matsumoto T, Nagai H, Banno T (1987) Observation of CSF pulsatile flow in MRI: the signal void phenomenon. Brain and Nerve 39:991–996 (English abstract)

Ouchi T, Shiga I, Negishi T (1985) A case of partial agenesis of the corpus callosum. Journal of NMR Medicine 5:93–96 (English abstract)

Naidich TP, Zimmerman RA (1985) Common congenital malformations of the brain. In: Brant-Zawadzki M, Norman D (eds) Magnetic resonance imaging of the central nervous system. Raven Press, New York, pp131–150

Naidich TP, Maravilla K, McLone DG (1986) The Chiari II malformation. In: McLaurin R, McLone D (eds) Proceedings of the Second Symposium on Spina Bifida. Grune and Stratton, New York

Naidich TP, Osborn RE, Bauer B, Naidich MJ (1988) Median cleft face syndrome: MR and CT data from 11 children. JCAT 12: 57–64

Novetsky G, Berlin L (1984) Aqueductal stenosis: demonstration by MR imaging. JCAT 8: 1170–1171

Nowell MA, Grossman RI, Hackney DB, Zimmerman RA, Goldberg HI, Bilaniuk LT (91988) MR imaging of white matter disease in children. AJNR 9: 503–509

Pennock JM, Bydder GM, Dubowitz LMS, Johnson MA (1986) Magnetic resonance imaging of the brain in children. Mag Reson Imag 4: 1–9

Pojunas K, Williams AL, Daniels DL, Haughton VM (1984) Syringomyelia and hydromyelia: magnetic resonance evaluation. Radiology 153: 679–683

Randt RS, Gebarski SS, Goetting MG (1985) Tuberous sclerosis with cardiogenic cerebral embolism: magnetic resonance imaging. Neurology 35: 1223–1225

Rock JP, Zimmerman R, Well WO (1986) Arachnoid cysts of the posterior fossa. Neurosurgery 18: 176–179

Roosen N, Gahlen D, Stork W, Neuen E, Wechsler W, Schirmer M, Lins E, Bock WJ (1987) Magnetic resonance imaging of colloid cysts of the third ventricle. Neuroradiology 29: 10–14

Roosen N, Schirmer M, Lins E, Bock WJ, Stork W, Gahlen D (1986) MRI of an aneurysm of the vein of Galen. AJNR 7: 733–735

Sakamoto M, Takeda K, Bandou M, Murayama S, Sakuta M (1985) A case of total agenesis of the corpus callosum: the diagnosis by NMR-CT and the localization of the speech center. Clin Neurol 25:454–457 (English abstract)

Samuelsson L, Bergstrom K, Thuomas K-A, Hemmingsson A, Wallensten R (1987): MR imaging of syringohydromyelia and Chiari malformations in myelomeningocele patients with scoliosis. AJNR 8: 539–546

Schindler E, Hajek P (1988) Craniopagus twins: neuroradiological findings (CT, angiography, MRI). Neuroradiology 30: 11–16

Scotti G, Scialfa G, Landoni L (1987) MR in the diagnosis of colloid cysts of the third ventricle. AJNR 8: 370–372

Sherman JL, Barkovich AJ, Citrin CM (1986) The MR appearance of syringomyelia: new observations. AJNR 7: 985–995

Sherman JL, Citrin CM, Barkovich AJ (1987) MR imaging of syringobulbia. JCAT 11: 407–411

Sherman JL, Citrin CM, Gangarossa RE, Bowen BJ (1986) The MR appearances of CSF flow in patients with ventriculomegaly. AJNR 7: 1025–1031

Shirakuni T, Tamaki N, Matsumoto S (1985a) Intracranial anomalies in myelomeningocele: observation with magnetic resonance (MR) imaging. Brain and Nerve 37: 481–487 (English abstract)

Shirakuni T, Tamaki N, Matsumoto S (1985b) Magnetic resonance imaging of child's brain. Part 3: lissencephalus. Brain and Development 17: 588–590 (English abstract)

Shirakuni T, Tamaki N, Matsumoto S (1986) Magnetic resonance images of central nervous anomalies. Adv Neurol Sci 30:474–485 (English abstract)

Spinos E, Laster DW, Moody DM, Ball MR, Witcofski RL, Kelly DL Jr (1985a) MR evaluation of Chiari I malformation at 0.15 T. AJNR 6: 203–208

Spinos E, Laster DW, Moody DM, Ball MR, Witcofski RL, Kelly DL Jr (1985b) MR evaluation of Chiari I malformations at 0.15 T. AJR 144: 1143–1148

Stimac GK, Solomon MA, Newton TA (1986) CT and MR of angiomatous malformations of the choroid plexus in patients with Sturge-Weber disease. AJNR 7: 623–627

Sze G, De Armond SJ, Brant-Zawadzki M, Davis RL, Norman D, Newton TH (1986) Foci of MRI signal (pseudo lesions) anterior to the frontal horns: histologic correlations of a normal finding. AJNR 7: 381–387

Tada S, Hata Y, Miyamoto Y (1985) Magnetic resonance imaging in craniovertebral junction anomaly. Jpn J Clin Radiol 30:340–344 (English abstract)

Tamaki N, Kojima N, Shirakuni T, Matsumoto S (1987) Arnold-Chiari malformation. Evaluation of its pathogenesis by magnetic resonance imaging, and surgical treatment. Neurol Med Chir 27:848–855 (English abstract)

Tamaki N, Nagashima T, Shirakuni T, Masumura M, Matsumoto S (1985) Magnetic resonance (MR) imaging in hydrocephalus: the pathophysiology of periventricular tissue. Progress in Computerized Tomography 7:255–264 (English abstract)

Tamaki N, Shirakuni T, Matsumoto S (1986) MRI of Arnold-Chiari type I malformation associated with syringomyelia (simple cylindrical type). Medical Postgraduate 24:436–439 (Japanese)

Tamraz JC, Iba-Zizen MT, Veres C, Cabanis EA, Godde-Jolly D, Braun M, Cosnard G, Laval-Jeannet M (1987) MRI in the central form of neuro-fibromatosis. 20 patients. J Neuroradiol 14: 365–382

Tanaka Y, Tabuchi M, Yamadori A (1985) Nuclear magnetic resonance (NMR) imaging of agenesis of corpus callosum. Neurological Medicine 22:596–598 (English abstract)

Thickman D, Mintz M, Mennuti M, Kressel HY (1984) MR imaging of cerebral abnormalities in utero. JCAT 8: 1058–1061

Tsukiyama T, Nishimoto H, Ogawa H, Kasahara E, Iwasaki M Tanaka O (1987) Magnetic resonance imagings of Alobar and semilobar holoprosencephaly. Nerv Syst Child 12:67–72 (English abstract)

Vaghi M, Visciani A, Testa D (1987) Cerebral MR findings in tuberous sclerosis. JCAT 11: 403–406

Venes JL, Black KL, Latack JT (1986) Preoperative evaluation and surgical management of the Arnold-Chiari II malformation. J Neurosurg 64: 363–370

Wiener SN, Pearlstein AV, Eiber A (1987) MR imaging of intracranial arachnoid cysts. JCA 11: 236–241

Wolpert SM, Anderson M, Scott RM, Kwan ESK, Runge VM (1987) Chiari II malformation: MR imaging evaluation. AJNR 8: 783–792

Yoshino A, Nishimoto H, Tsukiyama T, Komatsu A, Goto T, Shirata K, Tsubokawa T (1987) A bilateral huge middle cranial fossa arachnoid cyst in infant: with special reference to MRI-CT findings. Nerv Syst Child 12:471–478 (English abstract)

Yuh WTC, Barloon TJ, Jacoby CG (1987) Case report. Trigeminal nerve lipoma: MR findings. JCAT 11: 518–521

Yuh WTC, Segall HD, Senac MO, Schultz D (1987) MR imaging of Chiari II malformation associated with dysgenesis of cerebellum and brain stem. JCAT 11: 188–191

Zimmerman RD, Fleming CA, Lee BCP, Saint-Louis LA, Deck MDF (1986) Periventricular hyperintensity as seen by magnetic resonance: prevalence and significance. AJNR 7: 13–20

10 CNS Infections

The length of time required for an MRI examination is longer than that for CT. Since the procedure requires that the patient be absolutely still, considerable time may be required to calm him and get him to cooperate. Its use in acute conditions is thereby limited. The sensitivity of the MRI T_2 weighted image is a recognized advantage in inflammatory changes. In the T_1 weighted image, inflammatory changes are seen as areas of low to isointensity signal, but appear as high signal intensities on T_2. Hemorrhagic changes can also be shown more clearly on MRI.

Brain abscesses are clearly visualized on MRI, and vasogenic edema is particularly well depicted in the T_2 weighted image as a patchy low intensity shadow. It is not always possible to adequately demonstrate tuberculous meningitis, but enhancement of images by Gd-DTPA has been found to be useful. Herpes simplex encephalitis is well delineated by MRI. In the early stages, inflammatory changes located at the base of the frontal and temporal lobes are shown as a high signal intensity in the T_2 weighted image, appearing as patchy shadows. In the advanced stages of the disease, inflammation can be seen to extend from the central part of the temporal lobe to the insula and putamen.

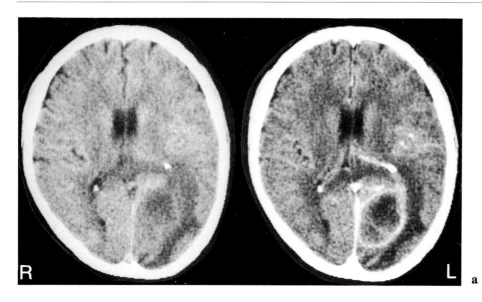

Fig. 10.1. Brain Abscess. A 68-year-old male. The patient presented with a history of fever (37.5°C) and headache of about 2 weeks' duration. He initially consulted a neighborhood clinic, where he was given treatment including antibiotics which provided some relief. A head CT scan was later done, revealing a left occipital mass and the patient was referred to our clinic. Upon examination, a right homonymous hemianopsia was found to be present.

a *CT scan.* A ring-enhanced mass with perifocal edema is seen in the left occipital region.

b, c *MRI.* The mass is shown as a low signal intensity in the T_1 weighted image and as a high signal intensity in the T_2 image. The extent of edema is well demonstrated in T_2. A thin capsule can also be seen in the periphery. A brain abscess was suspected and evacuation of the abscess was performed through burr holes.

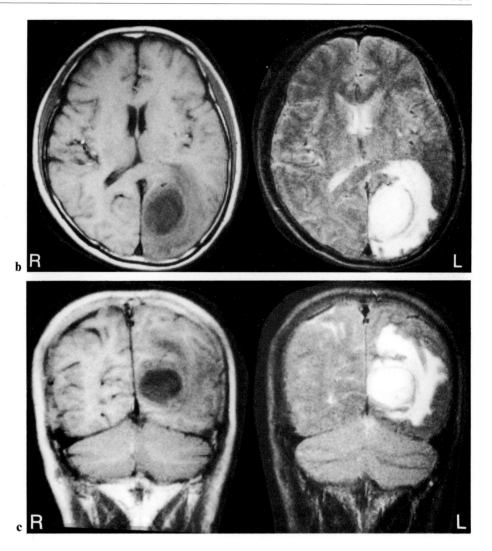

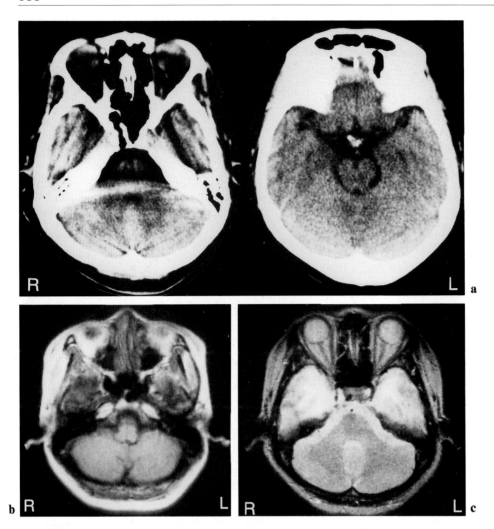

Fig. 10.2. Herpes Encephalitis. A 39-year-old female. The patient had had an attack of headache and fever 1 month prior to consultation. More recently, however, her speech had occasionally been incoherent, prompting her to visit our clinic. Upon admission, she was found to be disoriented. A lumbar puncture was performed with the following findings: opening pressure, 190 mmH$_2$O; CSF cell count, 656/3; monocytes, 99%; polymorphs, 1%, and HSV titer, 64 times.

a *CT scan*. A slightly low density area is seen in the right temporal lobe but is somewhat obscured by bony artifacts.

b, c *MRI*. High signal intensity areas are seen extending from the medial aspect of both temporal lobes to the hippocampus (greater on the right side) in the T$_2$ weighted image. There is no significant mass effect. The lesion was diagnosed as herpes encephalitis from the CT and MRI findings.

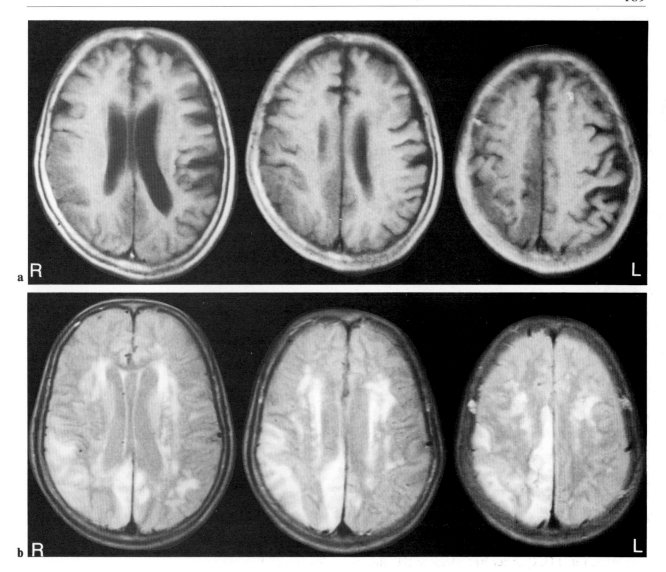

Fig. 10.3. Encephalitis. A 68-year-old female. The patient was brought to our clinic after falling down suddenly. On admission, she was comatose and had a left hemiparesis. Antibiotics were administered after a diagnosis of encephalitis was made, and she seemed to improve. A brain CT revealed no abnormality.

a, b *MRI*. There is a widening of the cortical sulci. In the T_1 weighted image, a cortical lesion, seen as a low signal intensity, extends across the parietal and occipital regions. The same lesion is seen as a high signal intensity in the T_2 weighted image. These features are consistent with those associated with encephalitis. High signal intensity spotty-to-patchy lesions are also seen in the periventricular area and putamen on both sides. Judging from the location of the lesions, an infarction is also suspected. Repeated MRI may give more information about the lesions — whether they are inflammations, edemas, fibroses, etc.

Bibliography

Atlas WS, Grossman RI, Goldberg HI, Hackney DB, Bilaniuk LT, Zimmerman RA (1986) MR diagnosis of acute disseminated encephalomyelitis. JCAT 10: 798–801

Davidson HD, Steiner RE (1985) Magnetic resonance imaging in infection of the central nervous system. AJNR 6: 499–504

Forman JM, Brownstone PK, Baloh RW (1985) Atypical brainstem encephalitis: magnetic resonance imaging and oculographic features. Neurology 35: 438–440

Grossman RI, Joseph PM, Wolf G, Biery D, McGrath J, Kundel HL, Fishman JE, Zimmerman RA, Goldberg HI, Bilaniuk LT (1985) Experimental intracranial septic infarction: magnetic resonance enhancement. Radiology 155: 649–653

Guilleux M-H, Steiner RE, Young IR (1986) MR imaging in progressive multifocal leukoencephalopathy. AJNR 7: 1033–1035

Gupta RK, Jena A, Sharma A, Guha DK, Khushu S, Gupta AK (1988) MR imaging of intracranial tuberculomas. JCAT 12: 280–285

Holland BA, Perret LV, Mills CM (1986) Meningovascular syphilis: CT and MR findings. Radiology 158: 439–442

Post MJD, Sheldon JJ, Hensley GT, Soila K, Tobias JA, Chan JC, Quencer RM, Moskowitz LB (1986) Central nervous system disease in acquired immunodeficiency syndrome: prospective correlation using CT, MR imaging and pathological studies. Radiology 158: 141–148

Post MJD, Tate LG, Quencer RM, Hensley GT, Berger JR, Sheremata WA, Maul G (1988) CT, MR, and pathology in HIV encephalitis and meningitis. AJNR 9: 469–476

Runge VM, Clanton JA, Price AC, Herzer WA, Allen JH, Partain CL, James AE (1985) Evaluation of contrast-enhanced MR imaging in a brain-abscess model. AJNR 6: 139–147

Schroth G, Kretzschmar K, Gawehn J, Voigt K (1987) Advantage of magnetic resonance imaging in the diagnosis of cerebral infections. Neuroradiology 29: 120–126

Suss RA, Maravilla KR, Thompson J (1986) MR imaging of intracranial cysticercosis: comparison with CT and anatomopathologic features. AJNR 7: 235–242

Zee CS, Segall HD, Rogers C, Ahmadi J, Apuzzo M, Rhodes R (1985) MR imaging of cerebral toxoplasmosis: correlation of computed tomography and pathology. JCAT 9: 797–799

11 Neurological Diseases

Since its introduction, MRI has been found to be clearly superior to CT in the diagnosis of degenerative changes, with lesions appearing as high signal intensity areas in the T_2 weighted image. The differential diagnosis of degenerative changes (including demyelination disorders such as multiple sclerosis and Binswanger's disease), and dysmyelination disorders (such as adrenoleukodystrophy and Alexander's disease) are best based on clinical findings, especially the patient's age and the course of the illness. Multiple sclerosis appears characteristically as patchy degenerations and is difficult to distinguish from infarction, although its relative symmetry may be helpful in the differentiation.

Spotty degeneration-like changes are often seen around the ventricles both in the elderly as well as in normal healthy persons. Care must be taken to avoid making an erroneous diagnosis of Binswanger's disease from the image alone. MRI differentiation is useful in the presence of dementia: in Alzheimer's disease, ventricles and sulci are dilated, and only cerebral atrophy is present. The presence of bony artifacts on the CT results in a poor demonstration of posterior fossa structures. These artifacts are absent on MRI, making it useful in the evaluation of degenerative changes of the cerebellum and spinal cord. In particular, the midline sagittal image demonstrates both the cerebellum and brain stem, and thus olivopontocerebellar atrophy (OPCA) or late cortical cerebellar atrophy (LCCA) can be diagnosed. In Parkinson's disease, the signal intensity of the midbrain and substantia nigra is reported to be low in the T_2 weighted image of high magnetic field MRI. However, this change is almost absent in MRI of less than average magnetic field strength.

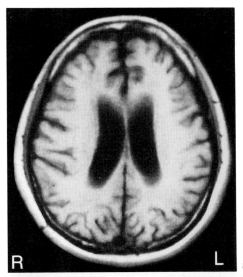

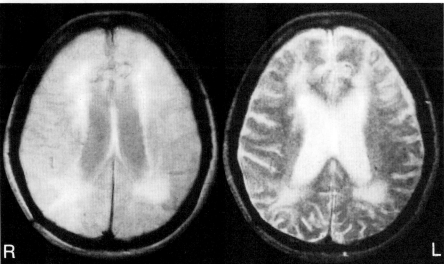

Fig. 11.1. Creuzfeldt-Jacob Disease. A 48-year-old female. The patient had a 2-year history of memory disturbance. One year ago, she also developed insomnia and the memory disturbance and disorientation became more severe. She underwent gradual impairment of function until the performance of simple tasks such as dressing and undressing herself became impossible. EEG showed frequent periodic single spikes dominant in the parieto-occipital region. No α-wave was noted with basic activity of low voltage irregular waves.

a, b *MRI.* Cortical atrophy and ventricular dilatation are visualized. Periventricular patchy high intensity lesions are present in the T_1 weighted image. Progressive cerebral atrophy is reported to be a characteristic MRI finding in this disease. Moreover, MRI makes it possible to detect intracerebral focal lesions and to demonstrate them three-dimensionally.

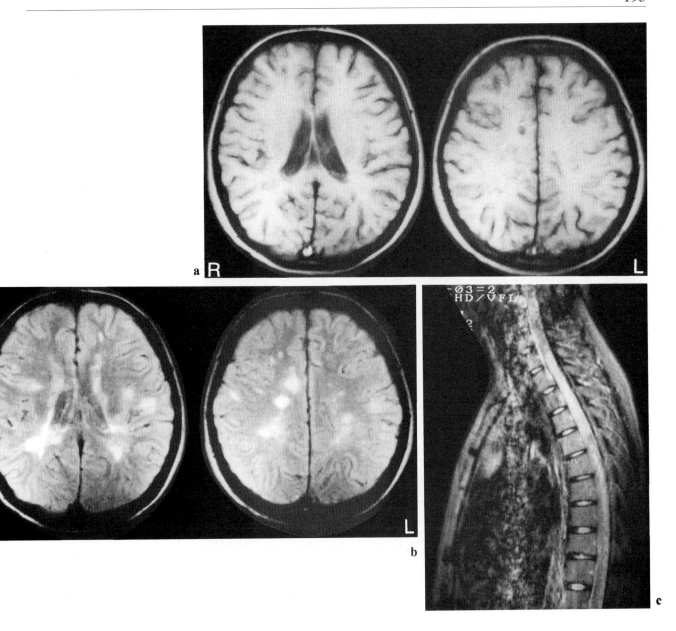

Fig. 11.2. Multiple Sclerosis. A 16-year-old female. The patient had a 2-year history of hearing disturbance in the left ear and visual disturbance of the right eye from which she later recovered. One year ago, she had a weakness of the right lower extremity which also disappeared after 1 month. More recently, however, the weakness of the right lower limb returned making it difficult for her to walk. At the time of admission, she was found to have sensory disturbance below the level of T5 and urinary incontinence. Babinski sign was elicited on both sides. The CSF IgG was increased to 11.8 mg/dl.

a-c *MRI.* A spotty-to-patchy high intensity is observed mainly in the periventricular region in the T_2 weighted image. A high signal intensity area is also seen in the T3–T4 thoracic cord. From the clinical and MRI findings, the diagnosis of multiple sclerosis was made.

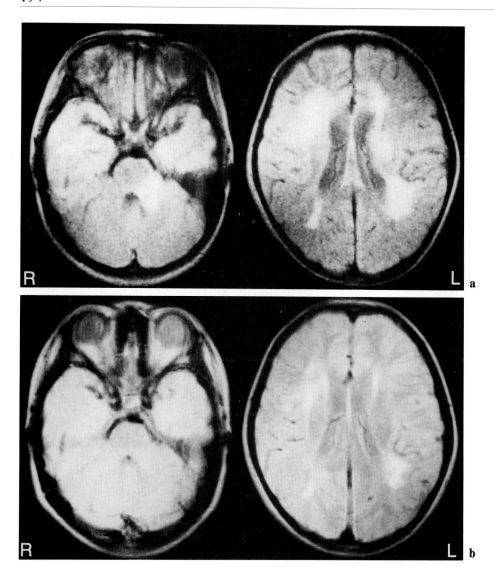

Fig. 11.3. Multiple Sclerosis. An 8-year-old female. The child had a seizure 3 months prior to visiting our clinic. Diplopia and blurred vision appeared 2 months later and she was evaluated by an ophthalmologist who diagnosed optic neuritis with left cerebellar signs.

a *MRI* (before treatment). Multiple patchy high signal intensity areas are seen in the left cerebellar peduncle, left basal ganglia, both insulae, and periventricular region.

b *MRI* (after treatment). Steroids were administered under a tentative diagnosis of multiple sclerosis. MRI performed 1 year after therapy shows the disappearance of lesions in the left cerebellar peduncle and left basal ganglia. The lesions in the periventricular area appear to have decreased. The cerebellar signs and optic neuritis have also improved.

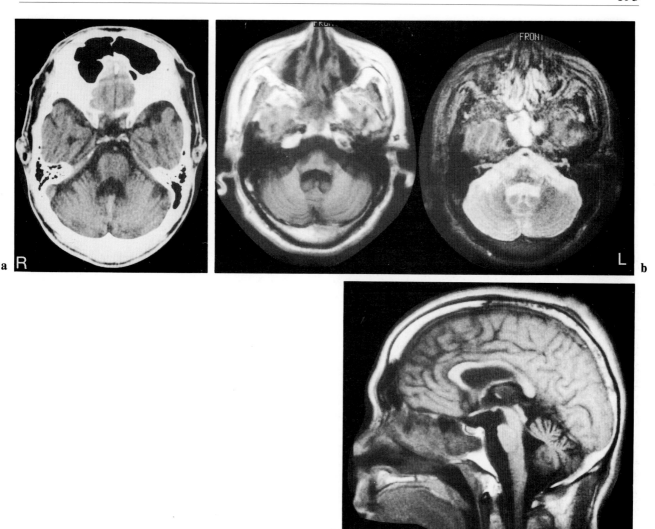

Fig. 11.4. Olivopontocerebellar Atrophy (OPCA). A 63-year-old male. There was a 1 year history of disturbance in gait and dysphagia and for the past 6 months the patient had difficulty in writing. A neurological examination revealed ataxic gait, cerebellar signs, slight rigidity, and a bilateral reduction of sensation for vibrations.

a *CT scan.* Marked atrophy of the cerebellum, pons, and medulla and dilatation of the fourth ventricle are seen.

b, c *MRI.* Similar findings to those in the CT scans are seen in T_1 (**b** left) and T_2 (**b** right) weighted images. Atrophy of the cerebellum and pons and enlargement of the fourth ventricle are well demonstrated in the T_1 weighted sagittal image (**c**). The diagnosis of OPCA was made from the clinical and MRI findings.

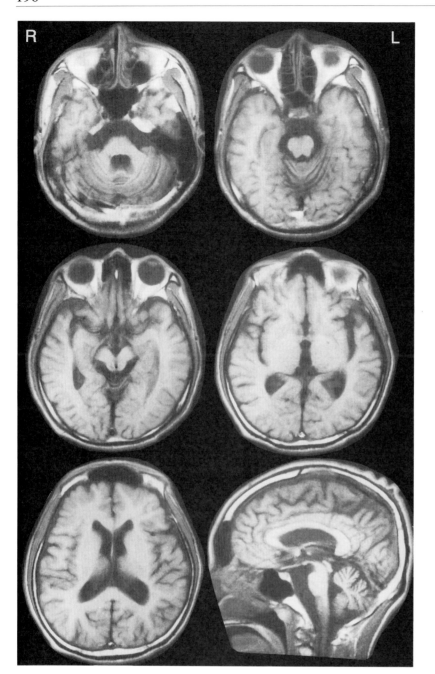

Fig. 11.5. Dentato-Rubro-Pallido-Luysian Atrophy (DRPLA). A 40-year-old male. The patient developed unsteady gait followed by speech and memory disturbances 15 years prior to consultation. Upon admission, he had an ataxic gait, cerebellar signs, and chorea-like involuntary movements.

MRI. There is atrophy of the whole of the brainstem, particularly in the midbrain and pontine tegmentum. There is associated dilatation of the fourth ventricle, and of the ambient and quadrigeminal cisterns. Both cerebral and cerebellar hemispheres also show atrophy. However, the caudate nucleus is normal. DRPLA was diagnosed based on the neurological and MRI findings.

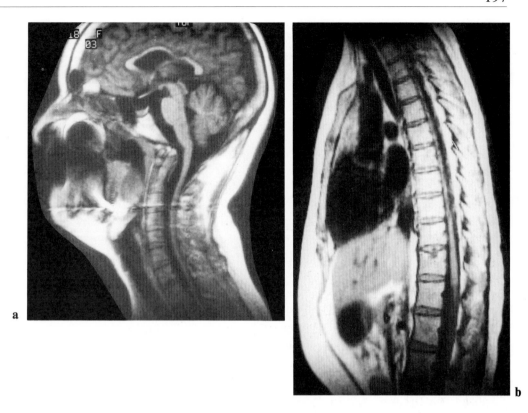

Fig. 11.6. Spinocerebellar Degeneration. An 18-year-old female. The patient presented with a history of disturbance of gait beginning at 13 years of age and progressing gradually thereafter. There was a past history of head trauma sustained in a traffic accident at that time.

a, b *MRI*. The spinal cord shows marked atrophy from the level of the upper cervical to the thoracic region. Atrophy of the cerebellum is not marked.

Bibliography

Aisen AM, Gabrielsen TO, McCune WJ (1985) MR imaging of systemic lupus erythematosus involving the brain. AJR 144: 1027–1031

Aisen AM, Martel W, Gabrielsen TO, Glazer GM, Brewer G, Young AB, Hill G (1985) Wilson disease of the brain: MR imaging. Radiology 157: 137–141

Atlas SW, Grossman RI, Goldberg HI, Hackney DB, Bilaniuk LT, Zimmerman RA (1986) MR diagnosis of acute disseminated encephalomyelitis. JCAT 10: 798–801

Baram TZ, Goldman AM, Percy AK (1986) Krabbe disease: specific MRI and CT findings. Neurology 36: 111–115

Bewermeyer H, Bamborschke S, Ebbardt G, Hunermann B, Heiss W-D (1985) MR imaging in adrenoleukomyeloneuropathy. JCAT 9: 793–796

Biller J, Graff-Radford NR, Smoker WRK, Adams HP, Johnston P (1986) MR imaging in "lacunar" hemiballismus. JCAT 10: 793–797

Brainin M, Reisner T, Neuhold A, Omasits M, Wicke L (1987) Topological characteristics of brainstem lesions in clinically definite and clinically probable cases of multiple sclerosis: an MRI-study. Neuroradiology 29: 530–534

Brant-Zawadzki M, Fein G, Van Dyke C, Kiernan R, Davenport L, Groot J (1985) MR imaging of the aging brain: patchy white-matter lesions and dementia. AJNR 6: 675–682

Burton K, Farrell K, Li D, Calne DB (1984) Lesions of the putamen and dystonia: CT and magnetic resonance imaging. Neurology 34: 962–965

Charness ME, DeLaPaz RL (1987) Mamillary body atrophy in Wernicke's encephalopathy: antemortem identification using magnetic resonance imaging. Ann Neurol 22: 595–600

Cherryman GR, Smith FW (1985) Nuclear magnetic resonance in adrenoleukodystrophy: report of a case. Clin Radiol 36: 539–540

Condon D, Patterson J, Wyper D, Hadley D, Grant R, Teasdale G (1986) Use of magnetic resonance imaging to measure the intracranial cerebrospinal fluid volume. Lancet 1: 1355–1357

Davis PC, Hoffman JC, Braun IF, Ahmann P, Krawiecki N (1987) MR of Leigh's disease (Subacute necrotizing encephalomyelopathy). AJNR 8: 71–75

De Witt LD, Buonmino FS, Kistler JP (1984) Central pontine myelinolysis: demonstration by nuclear magnetic resonance. Neurology 34: 570–576

Drayer B, Burger P, Hurwitz B, Dawson D, Cain J (1987) Reduced signal intensity on MR images of thalamus and putamen in multiple sclerosis: increased iron content? AJNR 8: 413–419

Drayer BP, Olanow W, Burger P, Johnson GA, Herfken R, Riederer S (1986) Parkinson plus syndrome: diagnosis using high field MR imaging of brain iron. Radiology 159: 493–498

Erkinjuntti T, Ketonen L, Sulkava R, Siponen JT, Vuorialho M, Iivanainen M (1987) Do white matter changes on MRI and CT differentiate vascular dementia from Alzheimer's disease? J Neurol Neurosurg Psychiatry 50: 37–42

Erkinjuntti T, Sipponen JT, Iivanainen M, Ketonen L, Sulkava R, Sepponen RE (1984) Cerebral NMR and CT imaging in dementia. JCAT 8: 614–618

Forman JM, Brownstone PK, Baloh RW (1985) Atypical brainstem encephalitis: magnetic resonance imaging and oculographic features. Neurology 35: 438–440

Friedland RP, Budinger TF, Brant-Zawadzki M, Jagust WJ (1984) The diagnosis of Alzheimer-type dementia. JAMA 252: 2750–2752

Fukuyama H, Kameyama M, Nabatame H, Takemura M, Nishimura K, Fujisawa I, Torizuka K (1987) Magnetic resonance images of neuro-Behcet syndrome show precise brainstem lesions: report of a case. Acta Neurol Scnad 75: 70–73

Gebarski SS, Gabrielsen TO, Gilman S, Knake JE, Latack JT, Aisen AM (1985) The initial diagnosis of multiple sclerosis: clinical impact of magnetic resonance imaging. Ann Neurol 17: 469–474

Gerard E, Healey ME, Hesselink JR (1987) MR demonstration of mesencephalic lesions in osmotic demyelination syndrome (central pontine myelinolysis). Neuroradiology 29: 582–584

Gomori JM, Grossman RI, Bilaniuk LT, Zimmerman RA, Goldberg HI (1985) High-field MR imaging of superficial siderosis of the central nervous system. JCAT 9: 972–975

Grossman RI, Gonzalez-Scarano F, Atlas SW, Galetta S, Silberberg D (1986) Multiple sclerosis: gadolinium enhancement in MR imaging. Radiology 161: 721–725

Guileux MH, Steiner RE, Young IR (1986) MR imaging in progressive multifocal leukoencephalopathy. AJNR 7: 1033–1035

Hata Y, Tada S, Uchiyama M (1988) Cerebral white matter lesions. Journal of Medical Imagings 8:391–397 (Japanese)

Holland BA, Kucharczyk W, Brant-Zawadzki M, Norman D, Haas DK, Harper PS (1985) MR imaging of calcified intracranial lesions. Radiology 157: 353–356

Horowitz AL, Kaplan R, Sarpel G (1987) Carbon monoxide toxicity: MR imaging in the brain. Radiology 162: 787–788

Huber SJ, Paluson GW, Shuttleworth EC, Chakeres D, Clapp LE, Pakalnis A, Weiss K, Rammonhan K (1987) Magnetic resonance imaging correlates of dementia in multiple sclerosis. Arch Neurol 44: 732–736

Iivanainen M, Hakola P, Erkunjuntti T, Sipponen JT, Ketonen L, Sulkava R, Sepponen RE (1984) Cerebral MR and CT imaging in polycystic lipomembranous osteodysplasia with sclerosing leukoencephalopathy. JCAT 8: 940–943

Jack CR, Mokri B, Laws ER, Houser OW, Baker HL, Petersen RC (1987) MR findings in normal-pressure hydrocephalus: significance and comparison with other forms of dementia. JCAT 11: 923–931

Kataoka S, Hirose G, Kosoegawa H, Oda R, Yoshioka A (1987) Brainstem type neuro-Behcet's syndrome: clinical correlation with brain CT and MRI. Clin Neurol 27:1025–1034 (English abstract)

Kawamura M, Shiota J, Yagishita T, Hirayama K (1985) Marchiafava-Bignami diseases: computed tomography scan and magnetic resonance imaging. Ann Neurol 18: 103–104

Ketonen L, Oksanen V, Kuuliala I (1987) Preliminary experience of magnetic resonance imaging in neurosarcoidosis. Neuroradiology 29: 127–129

Kinkel WR, Jacobs L, Polanchini I, Bates V, Heffner RR Jr (1985) Subcortical arteriosclerotic encephalopathy (Binswanger's disease). Computed tomographic, nuclear magnetic resonance and clinical correlations. Arch Neurol 42: 951–959

Kirkpatrick JB, Hayman LA (1987) White-matter lesions in MR imaging of clinically healthy brains of elderly subjects: possible pathologic basis. Radiology 162: 509–511

Kissel JT, Kolkin S, Chakeres D, Boesel C, Weiss K (1987) Magnetic resonance imaging in a case of autopsy-proved adult subacute necrotizing encephalomyelopathy (Leigh's disease)). Arch Neurol 44: 563–566

Kojima S, Kawamura M, Shibata N, Takahashi N, Hirayama K (1986) Magnetic resonance imaging of carbon monoxide poisoning in chronic stage. Clin Neurol 26: 291–299 (English abstract)

Kovanen J, Erkinjunti T, Iivanainen M, Ketonen L, Haltia M, Sulkava R, Sipponen JT (1985) Cerebral MR and CT imaging in Creutzfeldt-jakob disease. JCAT 9: 125–128

Kumar AJ, Rosenbaum AE, Naidu S, Wener L, Citrin CM, Lindenberg R, Kim WS, Zinreich SJ, Molliver ME, Mayberg HS, Moser HW (1987) Adrenoleukodystrophy: correlating MR imaging with CT. Radiology 165: 497–504

Laster DW, Penry JK, Moody DM, Ball MR, Witcofski RL, Riela AR (1984) Chronic seizure disorders: contribution of MR imaging when CT is normal. AJNR 6: 177–180

Leksell L, Herner T, Leksell D, Persson B, Lindquist C (1985) Visualisation of stereotactic radiolesions by nuclear magnetic resonance. J Neurol Neurosurg Psychiat 48: 19–20

Maravilla KR, Weinreb JC, Suss R, Nunnally RL (1985) Magnetic resonance demonstration of multiple sclerosis plaques in the cervical cord. AJR 144: 381–385

Miller DH, Johnson G, McDonald WI, MacManus D, du Bouley EPGH, Kendall BE, Moseley IF (1986) Detection of optic nerve lesions in optic neuritis with magnetic resonance imaging. Lancet 1: 1490–1491

Miller DH, Ormerod IEC, Gibson A, duBoulay EPGH, Rudge P, McDonald (1987) MR brain scanning in patients with vasculitis: differentiation from multiple sclerosis. Neuroradiology 29: 226–231

Minami M (1987) MRI diagnosis of demyelinating disease and degenerative disease. Neurological Surgery 15: 703–707 (English abstract)

Nabatame H, Fukuyama H, Akiguchi I, Kameyama M, Nishimura K, Nakano Y (1988) Spinocerebellar degeneration: qualitative and quantitative MR analysis of atrophy. JCAT 12: 298–303

Nishimura M, Fujita M, Kitahara Y, Akiguchi I, Kameyama M (1987) Magnetic resonance imaging in multiple sclerosis: the value of detecting lesions in periventricular white matter. Clin Neurol 27: 334–339 (English abstract)

Okazawa H, Inoue K, Yoshikawa K, Mannen T (1986) Magnetic resonance imaging of spinal lesions in multiple sclerosis. Clin Neurol 26: 1157–1164 (English abstract)

Oldendorf WH (1984) The use and promise of nuclear magnetic resonance imaging in epilepsy. Epilepsia 25: 105–117

Ormerod IEC, de Boulay EPGH, Callanan MM, Johnson G, Logsdail SJ, Moseley IS, Rudge P, Roberts RC, McDonald WI, Kendall BE, Macmanus DG, Ron MA, Zilkha KJ (1984) NMR in multiple sclerosis and cerebral vascular disease. Lancet 2: 1334–1335

Ormson MJ, Kispert DB, Sharbrough FW, Houser OW, Earnest IVF, Scheithaner BW, Laws ER Jr (1986) Cryptic structural lesions in refractory partial epilepsy: MR imaging and CT studies. Radiology 160: 215–219

Pastakia B, Polinsky R, Di Chiro G, Simmons JT, Brown R, Wener L (1986) Multiple system atrophy (Shy-Drager syndrome): MR imaging. Radiology 159: 499–502

Penner MW, Li KC, Gebarski SS, Allen RJ (1987) MR imaging of Pelizaeus-Merzbacher disease. JCAT 11: 591–593

Reider-Grosswater I, Bornstein N (1987) CT and MRI in late-onset metachromatic leukodystrophy. Acta Neurol Scand 75: 64–69

Rubinstein SS, Young AB, Kluin K, Hill G, Aisen AM, Gabrielsen T, Brewer GJ (1987) Clinical assessment of 31 patients with Wilson's disease. Correlations with structural changes on magnetic resonance imaging. Arch Neurol 44: 365–370

Runge VM, Price AC, Kirshner HS, Allen JH, Partain CL, James AE Jr (1984) Magnetic resonance imaging of multiple sclerosis: a study of pulse-technique efficacy. AJR 143: 1015–1026

Rutledge JN, Hilal SK, Silver AJ, Defendini R, Fahn S (1987) Study of movement disorders and brain iron by MR. AJNR 8: 397–411

Saida T, Fujisawa I, Nakano Y, Konishi T, Nishitani H, Torizuka K (1986) Magnetic resonance imaging of multiple sclerosis. Adv Neurol Sci 30: 486–494 (English abstract)

Schroth G, Gawehn J, Thron A, Vallbracht A, Voigt K (1987) Early diagnosis of herpes simplex encephalitis by MRI. Neurology 37: 179–183

Scotti G, Scialfa G, Biondi A, Landoni L, Caputo D, Cazzullo CL (1986) Magnetic resonance in multiple sclerosis. Neuroradiology 28: 319–323

Scotti G, Scialfa G, Tampieri D, Landoni L (1985) MR imaging in Fahr disease. JCAT 9: 790–792

Sheldon JJ, Siddharthan R, Tobias J, Sheremata WA, Soila K, Viamonte M Jr (1985) MR imaging of multiple sclerosis: comparison with clinical and CT examinations in 74 patients. AJR 145: 957–964

Shimoizumi H, Miyao M, Yamamoto Y, Kamoshita S (1986) Wilson's disease with peculiar MR-CT imaging. Clin Neurol 26: 631–635 (English abstract)

Simmons JT, Pastakia B, Chase TN, Shults CW (1986) Magnetic resonance imaging in Huntington disease. AJNR 7: 25–28

Simon JH, Holtas SL, Schiffer RB, Rudick RA, Herndon RM, Kido DK, Rosemary UTZ (1986) Corpus callosum and subcallosal-periventricular lesions in multiple sclerosis: detection with MR. Radiology 160: 363–367

Simon JH, Schiffer RB, Rudick RA, Herndon RM, (1987) Quantitative determination of MS-induced corpus callosum atrophy in vivo using MR imaging. AJNR 8: 599–604

Smith MA, Chick J, Kean DM, Douglas RHB, Singer A, Kendell RE, Best JJK (1985) Brain water in chronic alcoholic patients measured by magnetic resonance imaging. Lancet 1: 1273–1274

Soges LJ, Cacayorin ED, Petro GR, Ramachandran TS (1988) Migraine: evaluation by MR. AJNR 9: 425–430

Swanson PD, Cromwell LD (1986) Magnetic resonance imaging in cerebrotendinous xanthomatosis. Neurology 36: 124–126

Tadeka K, Sakuta M, Saeki F (1985) Central pontine myelinolysis diagnosed by magnetic resonance imaging. Ann Neurol 17: 310–311

Thompson AJ, Brown MM, Swash M, Thakkar C, Scholtz C (1988) Autopsy validation of MRI in central pontine myelinolysis. Neuroradiology 30: 175–177

Tjon-a-tham RTO, Bloem JL, Falke THM, Bijvoet OLM, Gohel VK, Harinck BIJ (1985) Magnetic resonance imaging in Paget disease of the skull. AJNR 6: 879–881

Udaka F, Kameyama M (1988) Clinical application of magnetic resonance imaging in neurology. Brain and Nerve 40: 423–437 (English abstract)

Waltz G, Harik SI, Kaufman B (1987) Adult metachromatic leukodystrophy. Value of computed tomographic scanning and magnetic resonance imaging of the brain. Arch Neurol 44: 225–227

Wilett J, Schmutzhard E, Aichner F, Mayr U, Weber F, Gerstenbrand F (1986) CT and MR imaging in neuro-Behcet disease. JCAT 10: 313–315

Yoshimura N, Nishizawa M, Hozumi I, Yuasa T, Miyatake T (1987) A case of leukoydystrophy, suspected of Alexander's disease, and its magnetic resonance imaging. Clin Neurol 27: 1141–1144 (English abstract)

12 Orbital Diseases

An external coil is often used when MRI of the orbital region is performed. The effectiveness of MRI in the orbit is comparable to that of CT, but MRI allows a freer creation of images and also demonstrates structures more clearly.

Melanomas and retinoblastomas are intraocular tumors. While melanomas generally affect adults, retinoblastomas are more common in children. Depending upon the melanin content, the signal intensity of melanomas varies; hemorrhage, which often accompanies it, produces an even more varicolored image. Because melanin pigment is paramagnetic, melanin-abundant melanoma shortens both T_1 and T_2 than more common tumors. Thus, it is seen as a high signal in the T_1 weighted image and as a low one in the T_2 image. Under these circumstances, it becomes difficult to differentiate between methemoglobin and fatty tissue. Retinoblastoma tends to present a more heterogeneous picture by virtue of its necrosis, hemorrhage, and high content of calcifications.

In tumors of the posterior orbit, it is important to ascertain the relative position of the optic nerve. It is possible to differentiate between meningiomas and the material of the optic nerve itself. Meningiomas show various signal intensities, but this probably depends upon the degree of calcification. Because of their fat components, dermoids appear as a high signal intensity in the T_1 weighted image, making diagnosis comparatively easily. It is often difficult to differentiate between cavernous angiomas, neurinomas, and metastatic tumors.

The rapid blood flow in vascular lesions such as AVM and carotid cavernous sinus fistulae is shown as a signal void, and diagnosis is therefore easy. If blood clots accumulate in the AVMs, this signal void will disappear. Idiopathic inflammatory pseudotumors are common intraorbital lesions in adults. They are comparatively easy to diagnose clinically, and steroids are believed to be effective in their treatment. They appear on MRI as isointensity signals in both the T_1 and T_2 weighted images. In thyroid orbitopathy, ocular muscles are enlarged and intraorbital fat is increased; in blowout fractures, the displaced orbital fat and ocular muscles are well displayed. In retinal detachments, fluid collected beneath the retina accumulates a large quantity of protein, making it difficult to differentiate it from ordinary hemorrhages. Fundoscopy is useful clinically and MRI can be used primarily to differentiate it from neoplastic lesions.

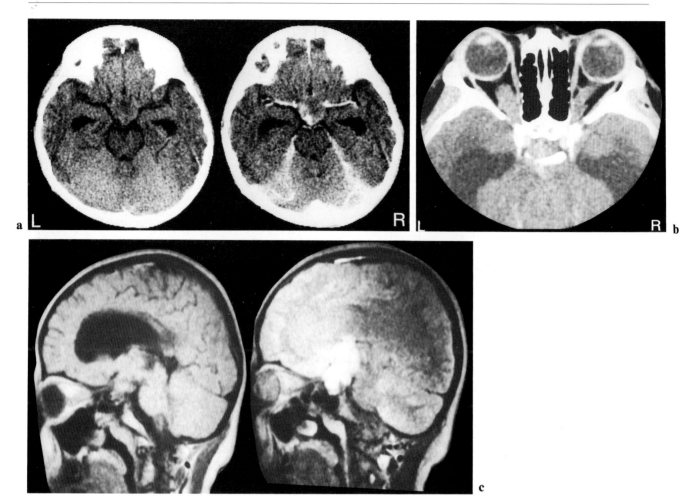

Fig. 12.1. Optic Glioma. A 12-year-old female. The patient came to our clinic with complaints of headaches and visual disturbances. Her visual acuity for the right and left eyes was 1.0 and 0.3, respectively, and could not be improved. There was also a defect in the upper left visual field. Fundoscopy revealed papilledema but there was no optic atrophy. No other neurological abnormalities were present, nor were there café au lait spots on the skin.

a, b *CT scan.* In the plain axial CT, marked dilatation of the inferior horn of the lateral ventricle and an isodensity mass are seen in the left optic nerve and hypothalamic region. The left suprasellar portion of the mass is enhanced in the contrast CT scan.

c *MRI.* In the T₁ weighted sagittal image, swelling of the left optic nerve and an isointensity mass are clearly demonstrated. In the T₂ weighted image, the mass is seen as a high intensity.

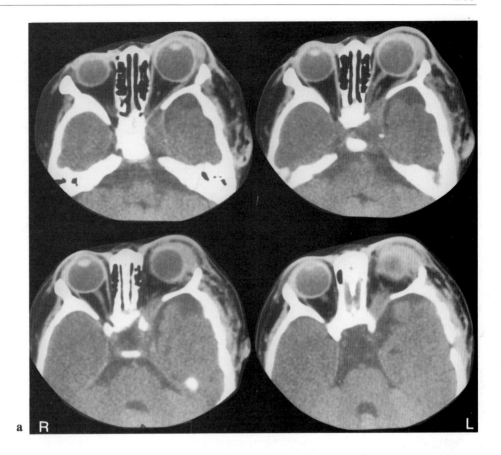

Fig. 12.2. Neurofibroma of the Orbit. A 2-year-old male. At birth the baby was noted to have 9 café au lait spots on the trunk. On a visit to a doctor for a common respiratory problem a left exophthalmos was noted and the patient was referred to our clinic.

a *CT scan.* The lesser wing of the left sphenoid is hypoplastic with marked left exophthalmos. A mass can be seen within and outside the muscle cone.

b–d *MRI.* The mass is seen in the left cavernous sinus superior to the orbit and extends over the orbit pushing it anterolaterally. It is of isointensity in the T_1 weighted image but of a relatively low intensity in the T_2 weighted image, and compresses the optic nerve medially. The mass was removed through a pterional approach and the diagnosis of neurofibroma was confirmed.

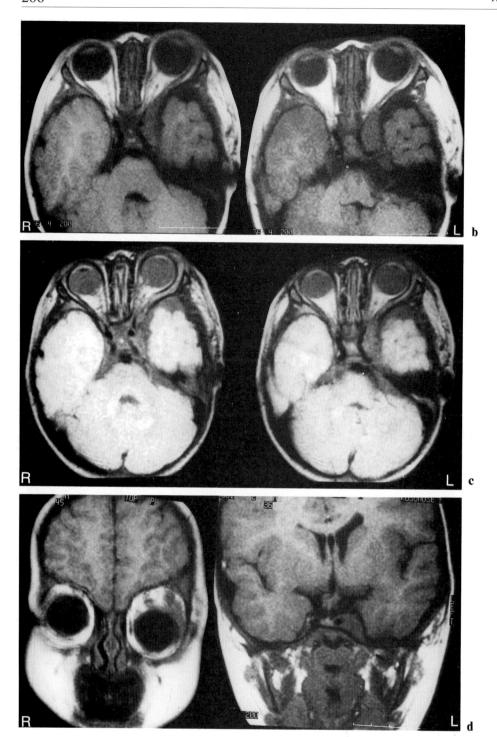

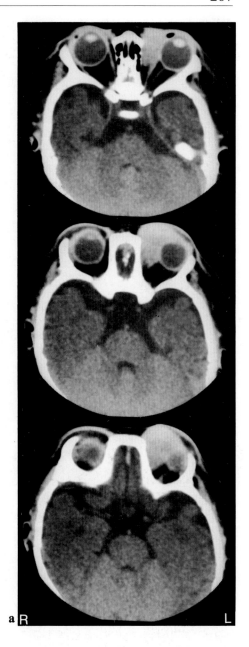

Fig. 12.3. Rhabdomyosarcoma. A 1-year-old male. Both the pregnancy and delivery were unremarkable. Four months after birth, the mother noticed a swelling in the child's left upper eyelid which gradually increased in size. He was brought to our clinic where a disturbance of the medial movement of the left eye was observed.

a *CT scan.* A large mass is seen medial to the left eyeball.

b, c *MRI.* The tumor, seen as an isointensity in the T_1 weighted image and as a high intensity in the T_2 weighted image, is located on the medial aspect of the left eyeball and depresses it inferolaterally. The tumor was removed and histologically confirmed to be a rhabdomyosarcoma.

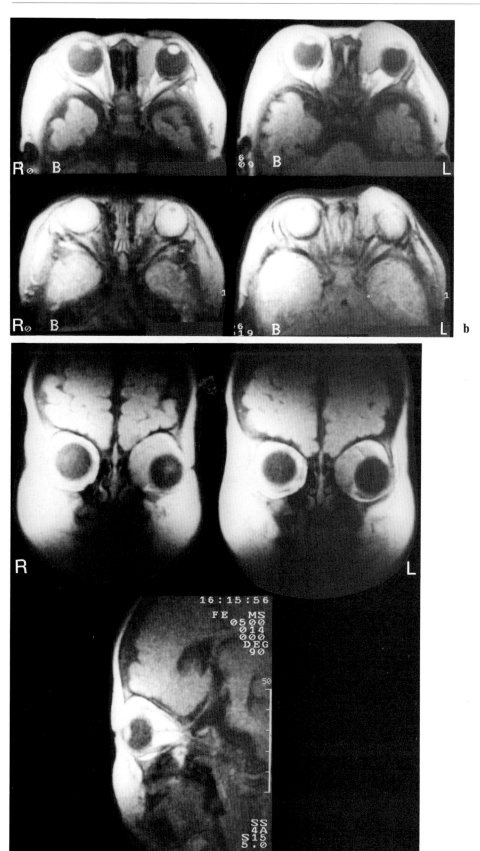

b

c

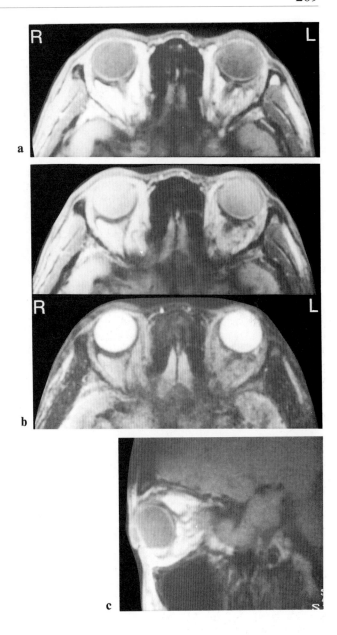

Fig. 12.4. Intraorbital Pseudotumor. A 50-year-old male. Left exophthalmos, swelling of the eyelid and diplopia developed several months prior to consultation with an ophthalmologist. The patient was referred to our clinic because an intraorbital tumor was suspected. There was no pulsation or bruit in the eye, and the eyeball movements were normal in all directions. There was double vision which was more marked on left lateral gaze. No endocrinological abnormality was discovered.

a–c *MRI*. In the T_1 weighted axial image (**a**), a poorly circumscribed inhomogeneous mass is seen between the optic nerve and the lateral rectus muscle. In the T_2 image (**b**), similar findings are also observed, but the high intensity component is more distinct in the T_1 weighted image. In the T_1 weighted sagittal image, the mass shows an isointensity.

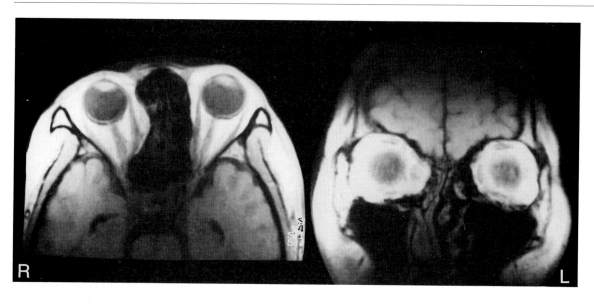

Fig. 12.5. Blowout Fracture. A 33-year-old male. The patient sustained an injury to his right eye.

MRI. The lamina papinacea of the right eye is destroyed, with the contents of the orbit bulging into the right ethmoid sinus in the form of a dome. There is invagination of the right internal rectus muscle into the right orbit and the diagnosis of a blowout fracture was made. MRI cannot show blowout fractures since it is unable to demonstrate bone. However, by virtue of MRI's good contrast of soft tissues, herniation of tissue within the orbit, especially extraocular muscles into the paranasal sinus or their shift is easily observed. Therefore, MRI is useful in determining which operative procedure is indicated.

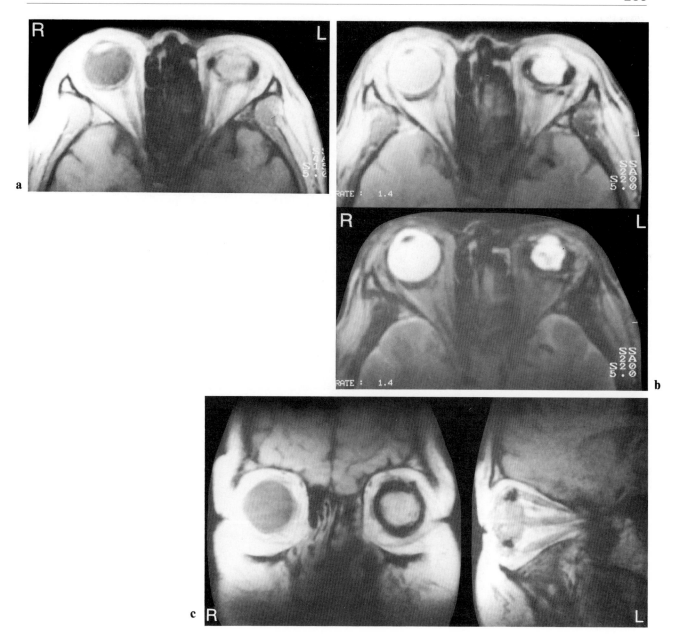

Fig. 12.6. Retinal Detachment and Vitreous Hemorrhage. A 32-year-old male. The patient sustained a blow to his left eye about 21 months prior to consultation. The affected eye is now completely blind.

a–c *MRI.* The anterior chamber and vitreous body are shown as a high intensity, and inside the eyeball an inhomogeneous structure with a mixture of isointensity is seen in the T_1 weighted image. In the T_2 weighted image, the eyeball is seen as a remarkably high intensity and contains a septum-like structure within it. These findings suggest the presence of retinal and vitreous hemorrhages. The left eyeball is atrophic in comparison with the right one.

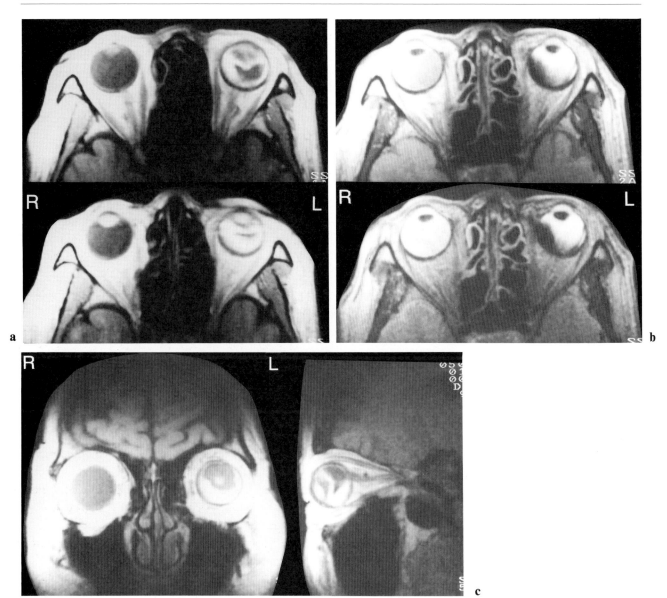

Fig. 12.7. Old Hemorrhage of the Vitreous Body. A 74-year-old male.

a–c *MRI.* An irregular abnormal intensity is seen in the vitreous body. The anterior portion of the vitreous body is seen as a high signal intensity in both the T_1 and T_2 weighted images, which probably represents extracellular hemoglobin. The posterior portion shows a high intensity in the T_1 weighted image and a low intensity in the T_2 weighted image, suggesting the presence of intracellular methemoglobin or a melanoma.

Bibliography

Atlas SW, Grossman RI, Savino JP, Sergott RC, Schatz NJ, Bosley TM, Hackney DB, Goldberg HI, Bilaniuk LT, Zimmerman RA (1987) Surface coil MR of orbital pseudotumor. AJNR 8: 141–146

Bilaniuk LT, Shenck JF, Zimmerman RA, Hart HR Jr, Foster TH, Edelstein WA, Goldberg HI, Grossman RI (1985) Ocular and orbital lesions: surface coil MR imaging. Radiology 156: 669–674

Char DH, Sobel D, Kelly WM, Kjos BO, Norman D (1985) Magnetic resonance scanning in orbital tumor diagnosis. Ophthalmology 92: 1305–1310

de Keizer RJW, Vielvoye GJ, de Wolff-Rouendaal D (1986) Nuclear magnetic resonance imaging of intraocular tumors. Am J Ophthalmol 102: 438–441

Dua HS, Smith FW, Singh AK, Forrester JV (1987) Diagnosis of orbital myositis by nuclear magnetic resonance imaging. Br J Ophthalmol 71: 54–57

Edwards JH, Hyman RA, Vacirca SJ, Boxer MA, Packer S, Kaufman IH, Stein HL (1985) 0.6 T magnetic resonance imaging of the orbit. AJR 144: 1015–1020

Fries PD, Char DH, Norman D (1987) MR imaging of orbital cavernous hemangioma. JCAT 11: 418–421

Gomori JM, Grossman RJ, Shields JA, Augsburger JJ, Joseph PM, De Simeone D, BSRT (1986) Choroidal melanomas: correlation of NMR spectroscopy and MR imaging. Radiology 158: 443–445

Jinkins JR (1987) The optic neurogram: evaluation of CSF "block" caused by compressive lesions at the optic canal. AJNR 8: 135–140

Johnson G, Miller DG, MacManus D, Tofts PS, Barnes D, du Boulay EPGH, McDonald WI (1987) STIR sequences in NMR imaging of the optic nerve. Neuroradiology 29: 238–245

Kato T, Sawada S, Shikaura S, Uda N, Kawa S, Tanaka Y, Miki H, Yamanouchi Y, Inagaki R (1988) MR imaging of orbital blow-out fractures. Progress in Computerized Tomography 10: 93–97 (English abstract)

Kelly WM, Paglen PG, Pearson JA, San Diego AG, Soloman MA (1986) Ferromagnetism of intraocular foreign body causes unilateral blindness after MR study. AJNR 7: 743–245

Li KC, Poon PY, Hinton P, Williansky R, Pavlin CJ, Hurwitz JJ, Buncic J, Henkelman RM (1984) MR imaging of orbital tumors with CT and ultrasound correlations. JCAT 8: 1039–1047

Lloydd GAS (1987) The orbit and eye. In: Sutton D (ed) A textbook of radiology and imaging, 5th edn. Churchill Livingstone, Edinburgh, pp1316–1841

Mafee MF, Peyman GA, Grisolano JE, Fletcher ME, Spigos DG, Wehrli FW, Rasouli F, Capek V (1986) Malignant uveal melanoma and simulating lesions: MR imaging evaluation. Radiology 160: 733–780

McArdle CB, Amparo EG, Mirfaohraee M (1986) MR imaging of orbital blow-out fractures. JCAT 10: 116–119

Okabe H, Kiyosawa M, Mizuno K, Yamada S, Yamada K, (1986) Nuclear magnetic resonance imaging of subretinal fluid. Am J Opthalmol 102: 640–646

Shenck JF, Hart HR Jr, Foster TH, Edelstein WA, Bottomley PA, Redington RW, Hardy CJ, Zimmerman RA, Bilaniuk LT (1985) Improved MR imaging of the orbit at 1.5 T with surface coils. AJNR 6: 193–196

Smith FW, Cherryman GR, Singh AK, Forrester JV (1985) Nuclear magnetic resonance tomography of the orbit at 3.4 MHz. Br J Radiol 58: 947–957

Sobel DF, Kelly W, Kjos BO, Char D, Brant-Zawadzki M, Norman D (1985) MR imaging of orbital and ocular disease. AJNR 6: 259–264

Sobel DF, Mills C, Char DH, Norman D, Brant-Zawadzki M, Kaufman L, Crooks L (1984) NMR of the normal and pathologic eye and orbit. AJNR 5: 345–350

Sobel DF, Moseley IF, Brant-Zawadzki M (1986) Magnetic resonance imaging (MRI) of the eye and orbit. In: Gonzalez CF, Becker MR, Flanagan JC (eds) Diagnostic imaging in ophthalmology. Springer, Berlin, pp99–118

Sullivan JA, Harms SE (1986) Surface coil MR imaging of orbital neoplasms. AJNR 7: 29–34

Zimmerman RA, Bilaniuk LT, Hackney DB, Goldberg HI, Grossman RI (1987) Paranasal sinus hemorrhage: evaluation with MR imaging. Radiology 162: 499–508

13 Diseases of the Spine and Spinal Cord

The spinal canal is a narrow space formed by bony elements including the vertebrae and vertebral discs, and extends from above downwards. Consequently, lesions in this region are characterized by longitudinal expansion in addition to lateral growth. With the development of the CT scan, methods for diagnosis of intraspinal lesions improved remarkably. However, because of bony artifacts and the fact that the longitudinal extent of lesions cannot be properly depicted, myelography is still used in addition to the CT scan. MRI, however, simultaneously provides the solution to all of these problems. Sagittal sections of the spinal column have become possible, making it easy to diagnose disorders of the spine, including spinal spondylosis, disc hernias, fractures, calcification of the posterior longitudinal ligaments, cancers, and spinal metastases. Diagnosis of diseases of the spinal cord, particularly those localized in the medullocervical cord junction and cervical cord has been greatly facilitated.

In reading the MRI, it is essential to know normal tissue structure and composition. The vertebral medulla is formed by bone marrow and fat, and the bone cortex is compact and contains an extremely small amount of free water. Thus, in the T_1 weighted image, the former is shown as a bright gray signal intensity, and the latter as a dark linear shadow. In older persons as well as in patients who have received radiotherapy, the spine presents as a higher signal intensity due to the increased fat content of the marrow. The intervertebral discs are generally seen as slightly lower signal intensity than the vertebral medullae. In the T_1 weighted image, cortical bones, ligaments and dural structures appear as low signal intensity and it is difficult to differentiate between them. Below L2, the intradural signal intensity is low due to the presence of CSF. However, in the low signal intensity area of the subarachnoid space in the cervical and thoracic regions, the shape of the spinal cord (which has a slightly lower signal intensity than the vertebral medulla) can be clearly recognized. The extradural space is wide posteriorly in the thoracic spine and anteriorly in the lumbosacral spine; because of the fatty tissue it contains, it appears as a high signal.

In the T_2 weighted image, the signal intensity of the spinal cord is low and that of the intervertebral disc is high, contrary to the findings on T_1 weighting. The high signal intensity of the disc is due to the water content of its predominantly gelatinous structure. A linear low signal intensity can quite often be seen in the central part of the disc due to invagination of a thin layer of annulus fibrosus, a finding generally present in persons over thirty years of age. Unlike the T_1 weighted image, the cortex of the vertebra gives a high signal. Therefore, in the cervical and thoracic spines, the subarachnoid spaces and spinal cord are difficult to differentiate. With prolongation of TE, however, the increase in the signal intensity of the subarachnoid space makes it possible to differentiate it from the shadow of the spinal cord. Enhancement of the images of these lesions with Gd-DTPA is very useful in their establishing diagnoses — as it is within the brain. It is most essential in the diagnosis of intramedullary lesions. In examining the spine and spinal cord, it is necessary to be aware that the spinal cord is influenced by pulsation, respiration, blood flow, CSF movement, and other factors which complicate the demonstration of spinal cord or extramedullary mass lesions.

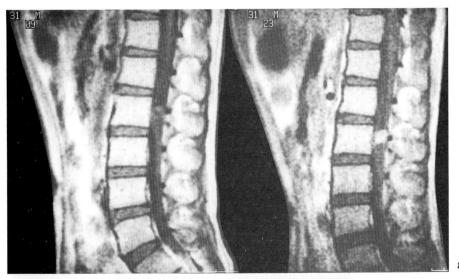

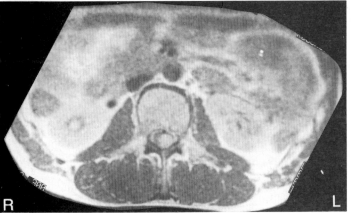

Fig. 13.1. Ependymoma in Conus Medullaris. A 54-year-old female. The patient
started to experience pain and weakness in the right lower extremity several weeks
before presenting at our clinic. There was also occasional urinary incontinence. A
neurological examination revealed flaccid paralysis, hypoactive deep tendon reflexes,
and sensory disturbance with the right being more markedly affected than the left.
The ankle jerk was normal on both sides.

a, b *MRI.* An iso to slightly high intensity mass is seen at the L2 level in the T_1
weighted image; it is well circumscribed with a high intensity in the enhanced scan.
In the axial image, the mass is located slightly to the left of the midline. The lesion
was diagnosed histologically as a myxopapillary ependymoma.

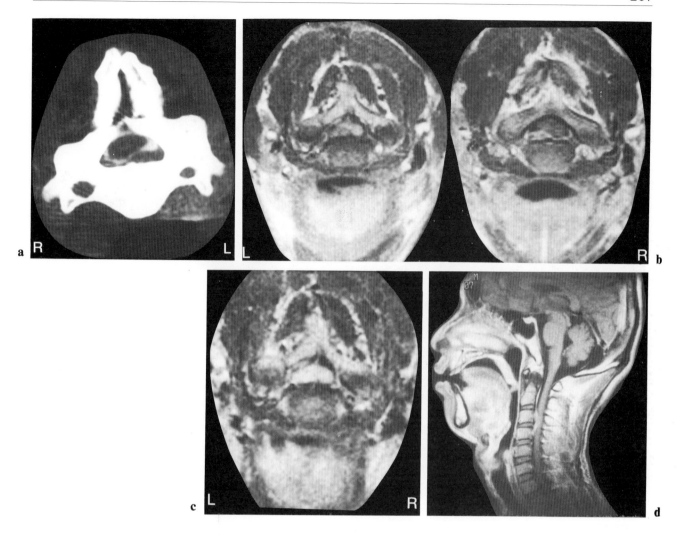

Fig. 13.2. Spinal Meningioma. A 40-year-old male. There was a 3-month history of pain in the occipital region and shoulder. Block therapy was administered several times, but since there was no relief, the patient was referred to our clinic.

a *Myelo CT.* The spinal cord is displaced posteriorly to the right.

b–d *MRI.* A dome-shaped mass is present behind the C3–C4 vertebral bodies which compresses and deforms the spinal cord. It is shown as an isointensity similar to that of the spinal cord, and the image is markedly enhanced with Gd-DTPA. The axial image shows deformity and posterolateral deviation of the spinal cord to the right. The diagnosis of intradural extramedullary tumor was made based upon the MRI findings. A tumor was removed subtotally by a posterior approach and confirmed histologically to be a meningioma.

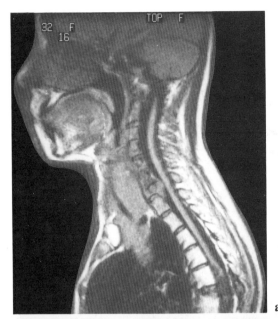

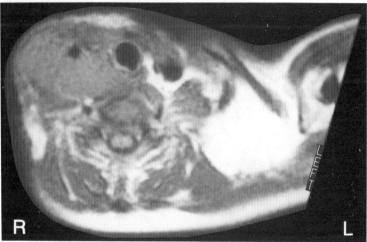

Fig. 13.3. Bone Metastasis from Thyroid Cancer. A 32-year-old female. A thyroidectomy was performed 3 years prior to consultation. One week before consultation, the patient developed numbness in both upper extremities. There was also a lymph node swelling on the right side of the neck.

a, b *MRI.* A mass measuring 6 × 4 cm is present in the neck and extends downward to the lung. The jugular vein is seen as a signal void spot in the central part of the tumor. A mass is also seen in the cervical vertebral body extending into the spinal canal. In the axial image, the tumor appears to extend posterolaterally on both sides, and either involves or compresses the nerve roots. T4 shows a compression fracture with loss of its original configuration. The mass invades the spinal canal and involves the spinal cord. From the above findings, it was felt that this was a case of recurrence of thyroid cancer associated with bone metastasis (C7–T6).

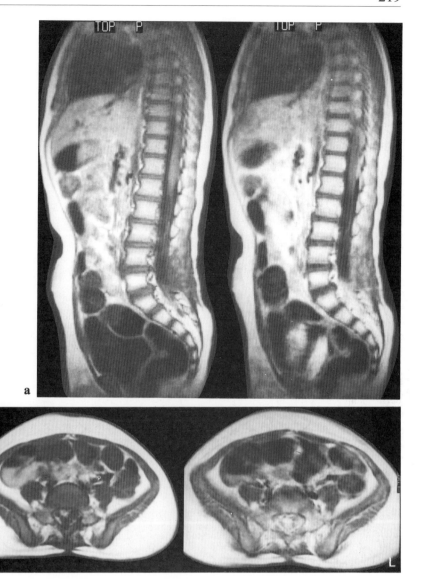

Fig. 13.4. Spinal Metastasis of Pineoblastoma. A 4-year-old male. Six months previously the child had undergone an operation for a pineal tumor which was histologically diagnosed as a pineoblastoma. Recently, he developed disturbances of gait and was said to fall down frequently. A neurological examination revealed weakness in both lower extremities and decreased knee and ankle jerks.

a, b *MRI*. An isointense mass which is enhanced by Gd-DTPA is present in the sacral segment of the spinal canal. From this finding, the diagnosis of spinal metastasis of pineoblastoma was made.

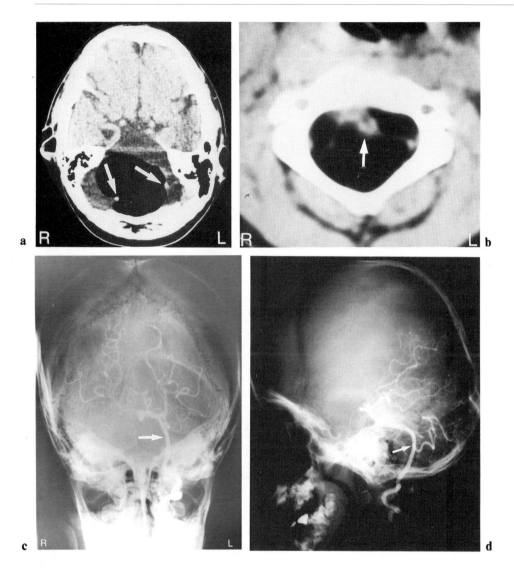

Fig. 13.5. Intramedullary Lipoma of the Cervical Cord and Posterior Fossa. A 7-year-old male. The child was delivered normally following a full-term and uneventful pregnancy. He was noticed to be tetraplegic soon after birth, which was believed to have resulted from a birth injury. At 5 years of age he started to have attacks of tonic-clonic convulsions in the left upper extremity. Upon admission, he was found to be incontinent, slightly mentally retarded, and had poor neck fixation. All four extremities were flaccid, and deep tendon reflexes could not be elicited.

a, b *CT scan.* A plain CT scan shows a large low density mass in the posterior fossa. Two high density spots (arrows) correspond to the vertebral arteries. The fourth ventricle cannot be identified. A CT scan of the cervical spine obtained after metrizamide myelography shows a high density area (arrow) corresponding to the cervical cord ventral to the low density mass.

c, d *Angiography.* Vertebral angiography shows a marked midline shift of the basilar artery to the left in the anteroposterior view (arrow). The basilar artery and the junction between the two vertebral arteries are displaced upwards and backwards, and the high position of the origin of the posterior inferior cerebellar artery (arrow) can be seen in the lateral view.

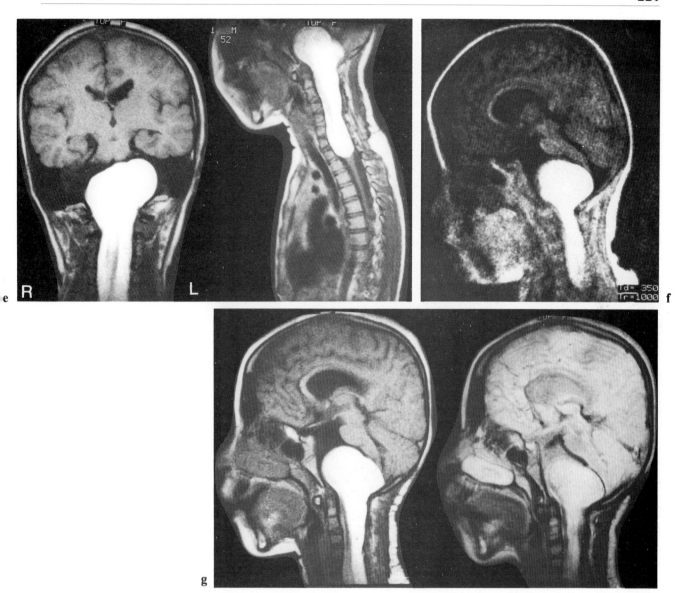

e–g *MRI.* The T_1 weighted image reveals an extra-axial mass ventral to the brainstem in the sagittal image. The fourth ventricle is identified lying posterosuperiorly to the mass.

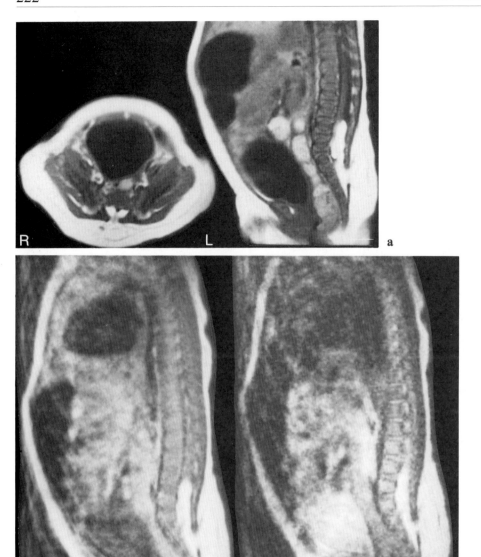

Fig. 13.6. Spinal Lipoma. A 2-year-old male. A mass was noted in the lumbar region to the right of the midline at birth. A physician to whom the child was taken because of a respiratory infection advised that specialist attention was required and referred the case to our clinic. A neurological examination revealed bilateral weakness of the lower extremities and slight weakness of the anal sphincter.

a, b *MRI.* In the T_2 weighted sagittal image, a high intensity mass is present in the spinal canal below L3 and part of it is connected with a subcutaneous mass of the same signal intensity. The spinal cord is adherent to the mass but does not protrude outside the spinal canal. In the T_2 weighted image, the signal intensity of the mass is lower. This finding is compatible with the presence of fat. The position of the cerebellum is normal and Chiari malformation is absent.

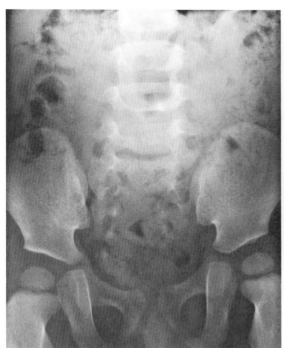

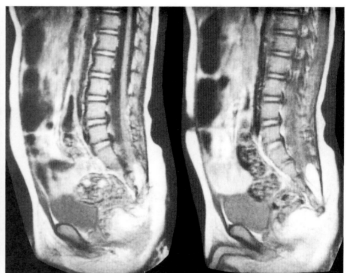

Fig. 13.7. Spinal Lipoma. A 1-year-old male. A mass was noticed in the coccygeal region at birth and the patient was referred to us with a tentative diagnosis of spina bifida. The neurological examination was unremarkable, but a definitive appendix was present in the coccygeal region.

a *X-ray of lumbosacral spine.* There is a widening of the interpeduncular distance at the level of L4 and below, but no apparent arch defect can be seen.

b *MRI.* A high signal intensity lipoma is seen in the sacral canal which is associated with tethered cord.

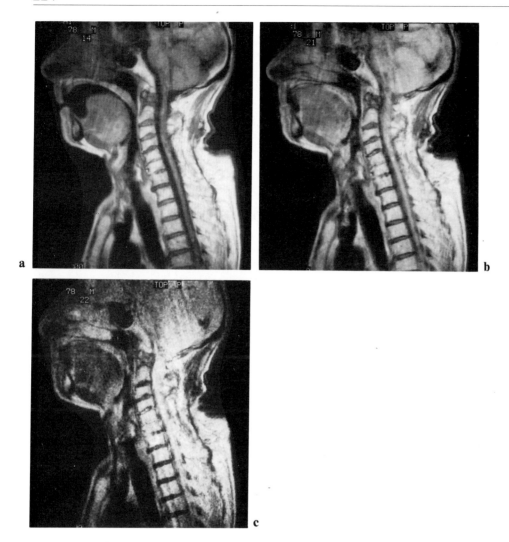

Fig. 13.8. Traumatic Cervical Cord Injury. A 78-year-old male. The patient sustained a neck injury and became tetraplegic 2 years prior to consulting our clinic. MRI was performed to evaluate the extent of the trauma.

a–c *MRI.* A low signal intensity is seen from C2–C5 in the T_1 weighted image; the same area appears as a high signal intensity in the T_2 weighted image. The C2–C5 segment of the cervical cord is swollen. The signal change is especially prominent in the C4–C5 region and suggests the presence of a traumatic myelomalacia. A narrowing of the disc space and spur formation are present and are most marked in the C5/6 and C6/7 areas. These changes suggest bone degeneration.

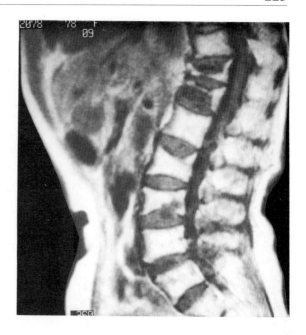

Fig. 13.9. Depressed Vertebral Fracture. A 70-year-old female. A few days prior to consultation, the patient fell down a flight of stairs and struck the back of her head against a hard surface. She experienced back pain which gradually became worse and which was later followed by numbness in the thoracic region. A neurological examination revealed a zone of hypesthesia in the T12–L1 area and tenderness of the back. Deep tendon reflexes were not exaggerated.

MRI. In the sagittal image, a depressed fracture is seen in the T12, L1, L3 and L4 vertebrae where there is shortening of the heights of the vertebral bodies and swelling of the discs. In the T12 and L1 vertebral bodies, a low intensity area due to hemorrhage is also seen. The normal vertebral body is seen as a high signal intensity. The lower signal intensity in the intervertebral discs may represent hemorrhage.

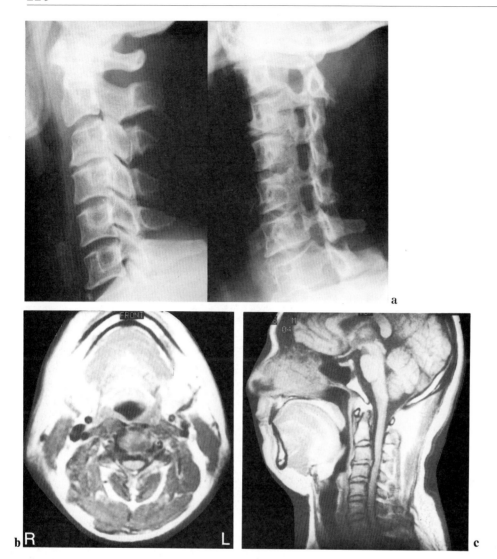

Fig. 13.10. Cervical Disc Hernia. A 48-year-old male. The patient had shoulder stiffness and headache for 1 year and more recently developed numbness in the fingers of both hands. He had been given a number of treatments including cervical traction and injections but the symptoms have failed to show any improvement. Upon neurological examination, slight atrophy of the deltoid muscles and an exaggeration of deep tendon reflexes were present on both sides.

a *X-rays of cervical spine.* A narrowing of the C3–C4 disc space and impaction of a bony spur into the intervertebral foramina are seen.

b, c *MRI.* Prolapse of the C3–C4 intervertebral disc is seen in the axial image. Compression of the spinal cord by the disc hernia is clearly demonstrated in the sagittal image.

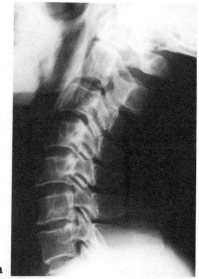

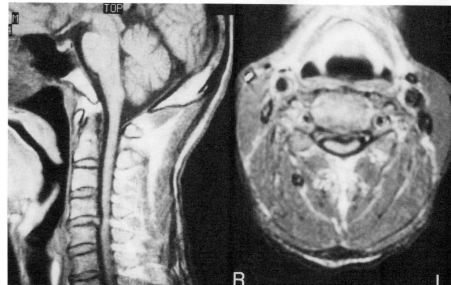

Fig. 13.11. Cervical Disc Hernia. A 56-year-old male. The patient noticed sensory disturbance of both upper extremities for about one year, and more recently noticed a reduction in his ability to grasp objects. Upon examination, dynamometry was 15 kg on the left and 30 kg on the right. Other findings compatible with myelopathy were also present.

a *X-ray of cervical spine.* There is a narrowing of the spinal canal with spondylotic changes.

b *MRI.* Posterior prolapse of the C4–C5 intervertebral disc is seen, and the spinal cord is compressed anteriorly by the prolapsed disc.

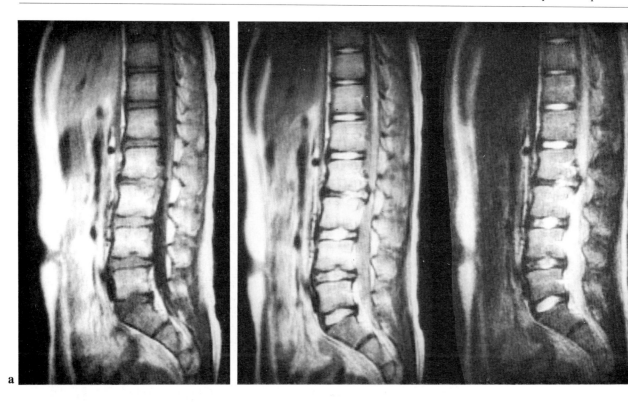

Fig. 13.12. Lumbar Intervertebral Disc Hernia. A 16-year-old male. The patient developed loin pain soon after a ball game but failed to receive treatment for it over the following 2 months. Lumbar pain gradually became more severe until the patient's gait became unstable and he was finally brought to our clinic.

a, b *MRI.* A narrowing of the disc space between L2 and L3 and posterior prolapse of the extruded disc material are present. The prolapsed disc markedly compresses the dural sac and spinal cord posteriorly and there is destruction of the vertebral chondral plates contiguous with the upper margin of L3 and the lower margin of L2 from the effect of the hernia.

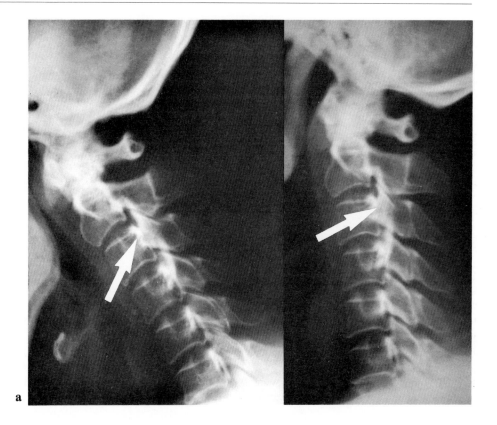

Fig. 13.13. Ossification of the Posterior Longitudinal Ligament (OPLL). A 50-year-old female. The patient had suffered from frequent attacks of shoulder stiffness in the past. One month before visiting our clinic she also developed disturbance in gait followed 2 weeks later by numbness and muscle weakness in the fingers of the left hand. Upon examination, the deep tendon reflexes in both the lower and upper extremities were hyperactive and there was sensory disturbance at the level of C5 and below.

a *X-rays of cervical spine.* Continuous ossification of the posterior longitudinal ligament can be seen (arrow).

b *CT scan.* An axial CT scan at the level of C3 shows a calcified mass behind the vertebral body. The spinal cord cannot be visualized.

c *MRI.* There is a signal void in front of the spinal cord at the level of C2–C4 in the sagittal image with compression and deformation of the spinal cord. Flattening of the spinal cord is well demonstrated in the axial image (arrow). Since bony structures give no signal on MRI, CT is superior in the demonstration of OPLL. However, spinal cord lesions are better demonstrated by MRI than by CT.

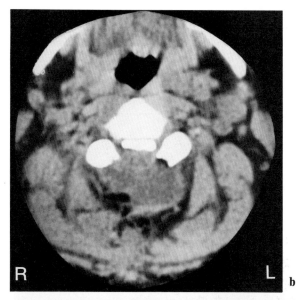

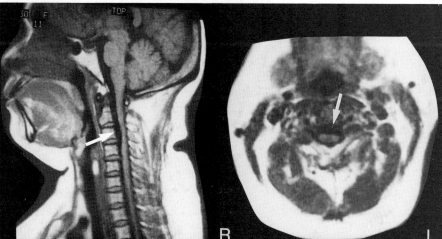

Bibliography

Aguila LA, Piraino DW, Modic MT, Dudley AW, Duchesneau PM, Weinstein MA (1985) The intranuclear cleft of the intervertebral disk: magnetic resonance imaging. Radiology 155: 155–158

Aii H, Koyama T (1988) Radiological imaging techniques in syringo-hydromyelia. Spine and Spinal Cord 1: 203–209 (Japanese)

Aichner F, Poewe V, Rogalsky W, Wallnofer K, Willeit J (1985) Magnetic resonance imaging in the diagnosis of spinal cord diseases. J Neurol Neurosurg Psychiat 48: 1220–1229

Aubin ML, Baleriaux D, Cosnard G, Cranzet G, Doyon D, Halimi P, Manelfe C (1987) MRI in syringomyelia of congenital, infectious, traumatic or idiopathic origin. A study of 142 cases. J Neuroradiol 14: 313–336

Barkovich AJ, Sherman JL, Citrin CM, Wippold FJ II (1987) MR of postoperative syringomyelia. AJNR 8: 319–327

Barnes PD, Lester PD, Yamanashi WS, Prince JR (1986) MRI in infants and children with spinal dysraphism. AJR 147: 339–346

Bertino RE, Porter BA, Stimac GK, Tepper SJ (1988) Imaging spinal osteomyelitis and epidural abscess with short T_1 inversion recovery (STIR). AJNR 9: 563–564

Bosley TM, Cohen DA, Schatz NJ, Zimmerman RA, Bilaniuk LT, Savino PJ, Sergott RS (1985) Comparison of metrizamide computed tomography and magnetic resonance imaging in the evaluation of lesions at the cervicomedullary junction. Neurology 35: 485–492

Braun M, Cosnard G, Cabanis EA, Iba-Zizen MT, Pharaboz C, Jean-Bourquin D, Derosier C, Perfettini C, Tamraz JC, Bocquet M (1986) NMR imaging and neuromas. J Neuroradiol 13: 209–225

Bundschuh C, Modic MT, Kearney F, Morris R, Deal C (1988) Rheumatoid arthritis of the cervical spine: surface-coil MR imaging. AJNR 9: 565–571

Burk DL, Brunberg JA, Kanal E, Latchaw RE, Wolf GL (1987) Spinal and paraspinal neurofibromatosis: surface coil MR imaging at 1.5 T. Radiology 162: 797–801

Bydder GM, Brown J, Niendolf HP, Young IR (1985) Enhancement of cervical intraspinal tumors in MR imaging with intravenous gadolinium-DTPA. JCAT 9: 847–851

Carsin M, Gandon Y, Rolland Y, Simon J (1987) MRI of the spinal cord: intramedullary tumors. J Neuroradiol 14: 337–349

Castillo M, Quencer RM, Green BA, Montalvo BM (1987) Syringomyelia as a consequence of compressive extramedullary lesions: postoperative clinical and radiological manifestations. AJNR 8: 973–978

Chafetz NI, Genant HK, Moon KL, Helms CA, Morris JM (1984) Recognition of lumbar disc herniation with NMR. AJNR 5: 23–26

Chakeres DW, Flickinger F, Bresnahan JC, Beatti MS, Weiss KL, Miller C, Stokes BT (1987) MR imaging of acute spinal cord trauma. AJNR 8: 11–18

Citri CM, Sherman JL, Gangarosa RE, Scanlon D (1987) Physiology of the CSF flow void sign. Modification by cardiac gating. AJR 148: 205–208

Crawshaw C, Kean DM, Mulholland RC, Worthington BS, Finlay D, Hawkes RC, Gyngell M, Moore WS (1984) The use of nuclear magnetic resonance in the diagnosis of lateral canal entrapment. J Bone Joint Surg 66b: 711–715

Daffner RH, Lupetin AR, Dash N, Deeb ZL, Sefczek RJ, Shapiro RL (1986) MRI in the detection of malignant infiltration of bone marrow. AJR 146: 353–358

Daniels DL, Hyde JS, Kneeland JB, Jesmanowic ZA, Froncisz W, Grist TM, Peck P, Williams AL, Haughton VM (1986) The cervical nerves and foramina: local coil MR imaging. AJNR 7: 129–133

Di Chiro G, Doppman JL, Dwyer AJ, Patronas NJ, Knop RH, Bairamian D, Vermess M, Oldfield EH (1985) Tumors and arteriovenous malformations of the spinal cord. Assessment using MR. Radiology 1566: 689–697

Di Chiro G, Knop RH, Girton ME, Dwyer AJ, Doppman JL, Patronas NJ, Gamsow OA, Brechbiel MW, Brooks RA (1985) MR cisternography and myelography with Gd-DPTA in monkeys. Radiology 157: 373–377

Dormont D, Assouline E, Gelbers F, Helias A, Halimi P, Chiras J, Bories J, Doyon D, Merland JJ (1987) MRI study of spinal arteriovenous malformations. J Neuroradiol 14: 351–364

Edelman RR, Shoukimas GM, Stark DD, Davis KR, New PFJ, Saini S, Rosenthal DI, Wismer GL, Brady TJ (1985) High-resolution surface-coil imaging of lumbar disk disease. AJR 144: 1123–1129

Enzmann DR, Griffin C, Rubin JB (1987) Potential false-negative MR images of the thoracic spine in disk disease with switching of phase- and frequency-encoding gradients. Radiology 165: 635–637

Enzmann DR, Rubin JB, DeLaPaz R, Wright A (1986) Cerebrospinal fluid pulsation: benefits and pitfalls in MR imaging. Radiology 161: 773–778

Enzmann DR, Rubin JB, Wright A (1987) Use of cerebrospinal fluid gating to improve T_2-weighted images, part I. The spinal cord. Radiology 162: 763–767

Enzmann DR, Rubin JB, Wright A (1987) Cervical spine MR imaging: generating high signal CSF in sagittal and axial images. Radiology 163: 233–238

Flanningan BD, Lufkin RB, McGlande C, Winter J, Batzdorf U, Wilson G, Rauschining W, Bradley WG Jr (1987) MR imaging of the cervical spine: neurovascular anatomy. AJNR 8: 27–32

Gebarski SS, Maynard FW, Gabrielsen TO, Krake JE, Latack JT, Hoff JT (1985) Post-traumatic progressive myelopathy. Radiology 157: 379–385

Gibson MJ, Buckley J, MaWhinney R, Mulholland RC, Worthington BS (1986) Magnetic resonance imaging and discography in the diagnosis of disc degeneration. J Bone Jt Surg 68b: 369–373

Glass RBJ, Poznanski AK, Fisher MR, Shkolnik A, Dias L (1986) MR imaging of osteoid osteoma. JCAT 10: 1065–1067

Goy AMC, Pinto RS, Raghavendra BR, Epstein FJ, Kricheff II (1986) Intra-medullary spinal cord tumors: MR imaging, with emphasis on associated cysts. Radiology 161: 381–386

Grenier N, Grossman RI, Schiebler ML, Yeager BA, Goldberg HI, Kressel HY (1987) Degenerative lumbar disk disease: pitfalls and usefulness of MR imaging in detection of vacuum phenomenon. Radiology 164: 861–865

Grenier N, Kressel HY, Schiebler ML, Grossman RI, Dalinka MK (1987) Normal and degenerative posterior spinal structures: MR imaging. Radiology 165: 517–525

Hackney DB, Asato R, Joseph PM, Carvlin MJ, McGrath JT, Grossman RI, Kassab EA, De Simone D (1986) Hemorrhage and edema in acute spinal compression: demonstration by MR imaging. Radiology 161: 387–390

Hackney DB, Grossman RI, Zimmerman RA, Joseph PM, Goldberg HI, Bilaniuk LT (1986) MR characteristics of iophendylate (Pantopaque). JCAT 10: 401–403

Hajek PC, Baker LL, Goobar JE, Sartoris DJ, Hesselink JR, Haghighi P, Resnick D (1987) Focal fat deposition in axial bone marrow: MR characteristics. Radiology 162: 245–249

Han JS, Benson JE, Kaufman B, Rekate HL, Alfidi RJ, Bohlman HH, Kaufman B (1985) Demonstration of diastematomyelia and associated abnormalities with MR imaging. AJNR 6: 215–219

Holtas SL, Kido DK, Simon JH (1986) MR imaging of spinal lymphoma. JCAT 10: 111–115

Jolescz FA, Polak JF, Ruenzel PW, Adams DF (1984) Wallerian degeneration demonstrated by magnetic resonance: spectroscopic measurements on peripheral nerve. Radiology 152: 85–87

Kan S (1988) Spinal cord lesions. Journal of Medical Imagings 8: 413–418 (Japanese)

Kantrowicz LR, Pais MJ, Burnett K, Choi B, Pritz MB (1986) Intraspinal neurenteric cyst containing gastric mucosa: CT and MRI findings. Pediatr Radiol 16: 324–327

Karnaze MG, Gado MH, Sartor KJ, Hodges FJ III (1987) Comparison of MR and CT myelography in imaging the cervical and thoracic spine. AJNR 8: 983–989

Kean DM, Smith MA, Douglas RHB, Martyn CN, Best JJK (1985) Two examples of CNS lipomas demonstrated by computed tomography and low field (0.08 T) MR imaging. JCAT 9: 494–496

Kim KS, Weinberg PE (1986) Magnetic resonance imaging of a spinal extradural arachnoid cyst. Surg Neurol 26: 249–252

Kokmen E, Marsh WR, Baker HL (1985) Magnetic resonance imaging in syringomyelia. Neurosurgery 17: 267–270

Kulkarni MV, Burks DD, Price AC, Cobb C, Allen JH (1985) Diagnosis of spinal arteriovenous malformation in a pregnant patient by MR imaging. JCAT 9: 171–173

Kunimoto M, Inoue K, Matsumoto A, Shimizu T, Mannen T (1987) The progress in radiological techniques and the change of the concept to syrnigomyelia: an analysis of 17 admitted patients for 20 years. Clin Neurol 27: 1372–1378 (English abstract)

Laakman RW, Kaufmen B, Han JS, Nelson AD, Clampitt M, O'Block AM, Haaga JR, Alfidi RJ (1985) MR imaging in patients with metallic implants. Radiology 157: 711–714

Lantos G, Epstein F, Kory LA (1987) Magnetic resonance imaging of intradural spinal lipoma. Neurosurgery 20: 469–472

Lee BCP, Deck MDF, Kneeland JB, Cahill PT (1985) MR imaging of the craniocervical junction. AJNR 6: 209–213

Lee BCP, Zimmerman RD, Manning JJ, Deck MDF (1985) MR imaging of syringomyelia and hydromyelia. AJR 144: 1149–1156

Lee M (1986) MRI of the spinal cord: especially the evaluation of syringomyelia, spinal cord tumor and spinal dysraphism. Adv Neurol Sci 30: 517–527 (English abstract)

Lewis TT, Kinsley DPE (1987) Magnetic resonance imaging of multiple spinal neurofibromata-neurofibromatosis. Neuroradiology 29: 562–564

Machida T (1986) Magnetic resonance imaging of the spine. Japanisch-Deutsche Medizinische Berichte 31: 43–49 (Japanese)

Mamourian AC, Briggs RW (1986) Appearance of Pantopaque on MR images. Radiology 158: 457–460

Maravilla KR, Lesh P, Weinreb JC, Selby DK, Mooney V (1985) Magnetic resonance imaging of the lumbar spine with CT correlation. AJNR 6: 237–245

Masaryk TJ, Boumphrey F, Modic MT, Tamborrello C, Ross JS, Brown MD (1986) Effects of chemonucleolysis demonstrated by MR imaging. JCAT 10: 917–923

Masaryk TJ, Modic MT, Geisinger MA, Standefer J, Hardy RW, Boumphrey F, Duchesneau PM (1986) Cervical myelopathy: a comparison of magnetic resonance imaging and myelography. JCAT 10: 184–194

Masaryk TJ, Ross JS, Modic MT, Boumphrey F, Bohlman H, Wilber G (1988) High-resolution MR imaging of sequestered lumbar intervertebral discs. AJNR 9: 351–358

Masaryk TJ, Ross JS, Modic MT, Ruff RL, Selman WR, Ratcheson RA (1987) Radiculomeningeal vascular malformations of the spine: MR imaging. Radiology 164: 845–849

Matsuoka Y, Machida T, Yoshikawa K, Iio M (1985) Magnetic resonance imaging of the tumor in the spine. Jpn J Clin Radiol 30: 1061–1067 (English abstract)

Matsuoka Y, Yoshikawa K, Machida T, Iio M (1987) Spinal cord disease and MRI diagnosis. Neurological Surgery 15: 813–818 (English abstract)

McArdle CB, Crofford MJ, Mirfakhraee M, Amparo EG, Calhoum JS (1986) Surface coil MR of spinal trauma: preliminary experience. AJNR 7: 885–893

Merine D, Wang H, Kumar AJ, Zinreich SJ, Rosenbaum AE (1987) CT myelography and MR imaging of acute transverse myelitis. JCAT 11: 606–608

Mikhael MA, Ciric IS, Tarkington JA (1985) MR imaging in spinal echinococcosis. JCAT 9: 398–400

Modic MT, Feiglin DH, Piraino DW, Boumphrey F, Weinstein MA, Duchesneau PM, Rehm S (1985) Vertebral osteomyelitis: assessment using MR. Radiology 157: 157–166

Modic MT, Masaryk T, Boumphrey F, Goormastic M, Bell G (1986) Lumbar herniated disc disease and canal stenosis: prospective evaluation by surface coil MR, and myelography. AJNR 7: 709–711

Modic MT, Masaryk T, Paushter D (1986) Magnetic resonance imaging of the spine. Radiol Clin N Amer 24: 229–245

Modic MT, Masaryk TJ, Mulopulos GP, Bundschuh C, Han JS, Bohlman H (1986) Cervical radiculopathy: prospective evaluation with surface coil MR imaginng, CT with metrizamide and metrizamide myelography. Radiology 161: 753–759

Modic MT, Masaryk TJ, Ross JS, Mulopulos GP, Bundschuh CV, Bohlman H (1987) Cervical radiculopathy: value of oblique MR imaging. Radiology 163: 227–231

Modic MT, Pavlicek W, Weinstein MA, Boumphrey F, Ngo F, Hardy R, Duchesneau PM (1984) Magnetic resonance imaging of intervertebral disc disease: clinical and pulse sequence considerations. Radiology 152: 103–111

Modic MT, Weinstein MA, Pavlicek W, Boumphrey F, Starnes D, Duchesneau PM (1984) MRI of the cervical spine. AJNR 5: 15–22

Monajati A, Spitzler RM, Wiley JLaR, Heggeness L (1986) MR imaging of a spinal teratoma. JCAT 10: 307–310

Mori K, Kamimura Y, Uchida Y, Kurisaka M, Eguchi S (1986) Large intramedullary lipoma of the cervical cord and posterior fossa. J Neurosurg 64: 974–976

Mukai E (1988) Magnetic resonance imaging in syringomyelia. Spine and Spinal Cord 1: 15–20 (Japanese)

Nabors WW, McCrary ME, Clemente RJ, Albanna FJ, Lesnik RH, Pait TG, Kobrine AI (1986) Identification of a retained surgical sponge using magnetic resonance imaging. Neurosurgery 18: 496–498

Okada E, Uyama E, Uchino M, Araki S, Koga K (1987) A case of intramedullary spinal cord hematoma with subacute transverse myelopathy which proved the usefulness of MRI. Clin Neurol 27: 1266–1269 (English abstract)

Okada Y, Matsuoka Y, Yoshikawa K, Machida T, Iio M (1987) Spinal cord disease and MRI diagnosis. Neurological Surgery 15: 929–933 (English abstract)

Okazawa H, Inoue K, Yoshikawa K, Mannen T (1986) Magnetic resonance imaging of spinal lesions in multiple sclerosis. Clin Neurol 26: 1157–1164 (English abstract)

Paushter DM, Modic MT, Masaryk TJ (1985)) Magnetic resonance imaging of the spine: applications and limitations. Radiol Clin North Am 23: 551–562

Pech P, Haughton VM (1985) Lumbar intervertebral disc: correlative MR and anatomic study. Radiology 156: 699–701

Pettersson H, Larsson EM, Holtas S, Croqvist S, Egund N, Zygmunt S, Brattstrom H (1988) MR imaging of the cervical spine in rheumatoid arthritis. AJNR 9: 573–577

Pojunas K, Williams AL, Daniels DL, Haughton VM (1984) Syringomyelia and hydromyelia: magnetic resonance evaluation. Radiology 153: 679–683

Quencer RM, Sheldon JJ, Post MJD, Diaz BD, Montalvo BM, Green BA, Eismont FJ (1986) MRI of the chronically injured spinal cord. AJR 147: 125–132

Ramsey RG, Zacharias CE (1985)) MR imaging of the spine after radiation therapy: easily recognizable effects. AJNR 6: 247–251

Rebner M, Gebarski SS (1985) Magnetic resonance imaging of spinal cord hemangioblastoma. AJNR 6: 287–289

Rodziewicz GS, Kaufman B, Spetzler RF (1984) Diagnosis of sacral perineural cysts by nuclear magnetic resonance. Surg Neurol 22: 50–52

Roosen N, Dietrick U, Nicola N, Irlich G, Gahlen D, Stork W (1987) MR imaging of calcified herniated thoracic disc. JCAT 11: 733–735

Ross JS, Perez-Reyes N, Masaryk TJ, Bohlman H, Modic MT (1987) Thoracic disk herniation: MR imaging. Radiology 165: 511–515

Rubin JB, Enzmann DR (1987) Imaging of spinal CSF pulsation by 2DFT MR: significance during clinical imaging. AJR 148: 973–982

Samuelsson L, Bergstrom K, Thuomas K-A, Hemmingsson A, Wallensten R (1987) MR imaging of syringohydromyelia and Chiari malformations in myelomeningocele patients with scoliosis. AJNR 8: 539–546

Sasaki M, Yamasaki Y, Higashida N (1987) A study of magnetic resonance imaging of the lumbar spine. Cent Jap J Orthop Traumat 30: 89–91 (English abstract)

Scotti G, Scialfi G, Colombo N, Landoni L (1985) MR imaging of intradural extramedullary tumors of the cervical spine. JCAT 9: 1037–1041

Scotti G, Scialfa G, Colombo N, Landoni L (1987) Magnetic resonance diagnosis of intramedullary tumors of the spinal cord. Neuroradiology 29: 130–135

Scotti G, Scialfi G, Landoni L, Pieralli S (1984) Nuclear magnetic resonance in the diagnosis of syringomyelia. J Neuroradiol 11: 239–248

Sherman JL, Barkovich AJ, Citrin CM (1987) The MR appearance of syringomyelia: new observations. AJR 148: 381–391

Sherman JL, Citrin CM, Gangarosa RE, Bowen BJ (1986) The MR appearance of CSF pulsations in the spinal canal. AJNR 7: 879–884

Solomon RA, Handler MS, Sedelli RV, Stein BM (1987) Intramedullary melanotic schwannoma of the cervicomedullary junction. Neurosurgery 20: 36–38

Steinmetz ND (1987) MRI of the lumbar spine. A practical approach to image interpretation. Slack, Thorofare NJ

Suojanen J, Wang A, Winston KR (1988) Pantopaque mimicking spinal lipoma: MR pitfall. JCAT 12: 346–348

Takahashi M, Sakamoto Y, Miyawaki M, Bussaka H (1987) Increased MR signal intensity secondary to chronic cervical cord compression. Neuroradiology 29: 550–556

Tashiro K, Ito K, Maruo Y, Homma S, Yamada Y, Fujiki N, Moriwaka F (1987) MR imaging of spinal cord in Devic disease. JCAT 11: 516–517

Teresi LM, Lufkin RB, Reicher MA, Moffit BJ, Vinnela FD, Wilson GM, Bentson JR, Hanafee WN (1987) Asymptomatic degenerative disc disease and spondylosis of the cervical spine: MR imaging. Radiology 164: 83–88

Thron A, Schroth G (1986) Magnetic resonance imaging (MRI) of diastematomyelia. Neuroradiology 28: 371–372

Valk J (1988) Gd-DTPA in MR of spinal lesions. AJNR 9: 345–350

Wilberger JE, Maroon JC, Prostko ER, Baghai P, Beckman I, Deeb ZL II (1987) Magnetic resonance imaging and intraoperative neurosonography in syringomyelia. Neurosurgery 20: 599–605

Williams AL, Haughton VM, Pojunas KW, Daniels DL, Kilgore DP (1987) Differentiation of intramedullary neoplasms and cyst by MR. AJR 149: 159–164

Yoshikawa K (1984) MRI diagnosis of spine and spinal cord diseases. Journal of Medical Imagings 4: 1119–1125 (Japanese)

Yoshikawa K (1985) MRI (magnetic resonance imaging) in the diagnosis of syringomyelia. Neurological Medicine 23: 16–23 (English abstract)

Subject Index